DOCTOR KARIN'S

COMBAT DIS-EASE SERIES

BOOK II

COMBAT

HEADACHES

BY KARIN V. DRUMMOND, DC

DOCTOR KARIN'S
COMBAT
HEADACHES

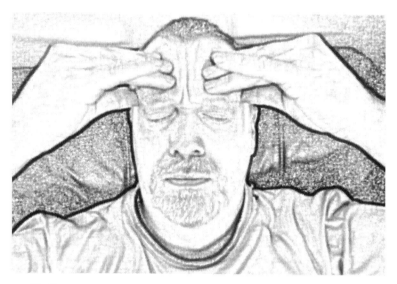

COMBAT DIS-EASE SERIES
BOOK II

A chiropractor's advice for those who suffer from migraines, jaw pain, sinus pain, and/or tension headaches without resorting to taking pain medication.

BY KARIN V. DRUMMOND, DC

Published by Blooming Ink Publishing, LLC

4712 East State Road 46
Bloomington, IN 47401

FIRST EDITION

ISBN 978-1-943753-04-8

Library of Congress Control Number: 2016905176

This book is dedicated to my patients and anyone who benefits from reading my books.

A special thank you to:
My family for being the foundation on which I stand.
Fine Art Images by George, LLC, for my image on the front cover.
Kip May Photography for my image on the back cover.
Josh Gonzalez with EarWig Design for designing my book covers.
Johanna Salazar and Rian Dawson for their editing skills.
Vicki Adang, my professional editor, for taking on this project.

And thank you to countless others…

**May this book be
my message in a bottle
in the sea of misinformation.**

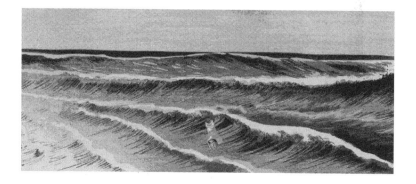

Preface

Dear Reader,

I assume that because you bought this book, you or a loved one is suffering from headaches, migraines, sinus pain, jaw pain, tension, or some other head pain. Rest assured, I wrote this book for you.

As a chiropractor, I have extensive experience with treating headaches. Over the years I have found myself giving patients the same explanations for causes and treatments every day. Now, not only can I can hand my patients this book to empower them to do many of the treatments themselves, but I can offer my advice and treatments to countless others who suffer the same pain.

In this book, I have explained how to determine what type of headache you're suffering from, provided examples of exercises and stretches to help recovery, outlined treatments to consider, and included advice on how to get better, including my personal thoughts on living well.

We are all individuals with unique conditions and needs, so I advise that you consult with a health professional for guidance before following the advice in this book.

I wish you or your loved one wellness and a speedy recovery.

Karin Drummond, D.C.

Dr. Karin's Definition of Dis-ease

Dis-ease is a state of being that results when a person is under prolonged stress, independent of whether it is a physical or mental stressor. Simply, it is a state of agitation and non-relaxation.

The human body evolved to handle physical stress: you either survive or you die. For example, if you get attacked by a tiger, your body automatically goes through steps to decide between fighting or fleeing. Your adrenaline kicks in, activated by your flight-or-flight sympathetic nervous system.

Blood flows out of your internal organs and into your arms and legs. This rerouting of energy and blood gives you extra strength and endurance, and decreases the amount of blood loss you would experience from your organs if you were to be wounded. Your primitive brain controls all of this automatically; you don't even think about it. Your only job is to act and survive.

The primitive brain cannot tell the difference between a mental and a physical stressor. Its reaction is the same: to prepare your body for fight or flight. But if your stressor is due to work or an argument with a loved one, the primitive brain's fight-or-flight response is disproportional to the threat of the stressor. Your body is prepared to move, but instead you sit, tense. This is unhealthy over time because the lymphatic system (the body's sewage system) requires movement to drain the metabolic waste out of your tissues.

If the muscles stay tense, they not only prevent lymphatic drainage, but also impair the blood flow to the very muscles being contracted. These constantly contracting muscles produce metabolic waste (lactic acid) and need the oxygen-filled blood to be able to contract, yet they are blocking the very flow of fluids that brings in their nutrients and drains their waste. This sitting tense and stressed out is unhealthy over time because it leads to the buildup of toxins in the body. This is one reason why stressed people tend to be tender to touch.

Prolonged stress leads to adrenal fatigue; if you need a boost of energy, your body just doesn't have it to give to you. Your digestive system suffers from the diminished blood supply (because the fight-or-flight response has diverted blood away from internal organs). Then your appetite changes as you become deficient in nutrients within the intestines, leading to either weight gain or excessive weight loss.

Your blood pressure also goes up as a result of oversupplying blood to your extremities for the anticipated fight or flight. Over time, your arteries harden from being under such high pressure in a low-nutrient environment.

Eventually, your body starts deteriorating, becoming more susceptible to sickness. Every day your body fights viruses, bacteria, and fungi as well as mutations in a few of your one hundred trillion cells. It starts to lose these battles when weakened by stress, thus becoming more susceptible to colds, allergies, flu viruses, infections, cancer, and other grave diseases.

All of these can result in a headache!

Stress is the number one cause of death; it's just given names like heart attack, cancer, stroke, suicide, etc.

This book addresses headaches, a symptom of being in a diseased state. Learn how stress and lifestyle affect your headaches.

This book and my other books have advice on how to break this vicious cycle of stress, which leads to pain, a sign of "dis-ease," which in turn can lead to physical disease and, potentially, an early death.

BE AT EASE,
AVOID DIS-EASE.

Contents

Chapter 1 : THE DIFFERENT TYPES OF HEADACHES

I WANT TO START the battle against headaches by describing the different types of headaches you may experience. Even though any of the treatments I describe in this book can generally relieve any type of headache, you need to understand why and how my treatment plans work. And being able to identify different types of headaches will help you determine which treatments are the most effective, in terms of both time and money.

Ultimately, the cure for any headache is not that complicated, but it may be difficult for some to follow. I hope to motivate you with the promise of success. Understanding the type(s) of headaches you suffer from will help you understand how the treatments work and will motivate you to follow the headache treatment regimen.

So, let's go over the different types of headaches (head pains).

Primary Headaches

Primary headaches are caused by irritation to the nerves

and/or inflammation of the blood vessels in the head. The most common type of primary headache is a tension headache.

Tension Headaches

Tension headaches are often described as the pain you would feel if you had a band wrapped around and squeezing your head.

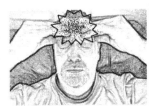

Roughly 90 percent of all headaches that I see are caused by tension. When muscles in the neck become tense, they pinch the nerves that send signals to the head. The most common tension headache is caused by pressure from tight suboccipital muscles on the greater occipital nerve (Figure 1-1).

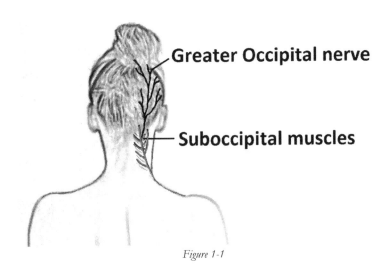

Greater Occipital nerve

Suboccipital muscles

Figure 1-1

To explain this phenomenon, I like to use a more commonly known medical condition, sciatica, as an example of how a pinched nerve causes pain in the part of the body that the nerve supplies.

The sciatic nerve sends signals down the back side of the thigh and through most of the lower leg and foot. Sciatica occurs when the nerve is irritated or inflamed. Such irritation can result when a muscle in the buttock pinches the sciatic nerve. Because the sciatic nerve only knows how to communicate input from the leg, when the nerve is pinched, it screams, "Severe leg pain!" to the brain. This is why when the sciatic nerve is pinched, a person feels severe pain that radiates down the leg.

Similarly, the greater occipital nerve only knows to communicate sensations from the head. So when it's pinched, it screams, "Severe head pain!" This is why I say that a tension headache is like having sciatica of the head (Figure 1-2).

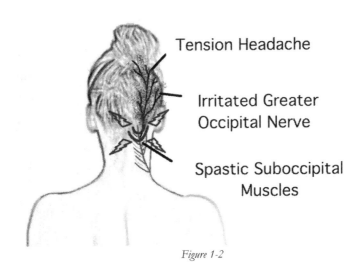

Tension Headache

Irritated Greater
Occipital Nerve

Spastic Suboccipital
Muscles

Figure 1-2

When the muscles at the base of the skull and top of the neck contract too strongly or sustain their contraction for a prolonged period of time (for example, slouching in front of a computer screen for hours), they squish the nerves supplying the head, causing a band of pain across the front of the head (where the nerves end).

People can also suffer from one-sided tension headaches. Leaning to one side while sitting for a long period, like when you rest your left arm on an armrest and use a mouse with your right hand, can lead to one-sided spasms of the neck's posterior muscles (the muscles in the back of the neck). A one-sided tension headache can mimic migraine headaches and lead to the misdiagnosis of tension headaches as migraines. This misdiagnosis may explain why migraine medication is not working for you.

Another cause of tension headaches can be muscle tension in

the front of the neck. This occurs when super-sensitive trigger points on the muscles cause people to feel pain into the head. Figure 1-3 shows the sternocleidomastoid and trapezius muscles, which have trigger points at the dots. When those trigger points experience too much pressure, they send pain signals to the sprayed area of the head.

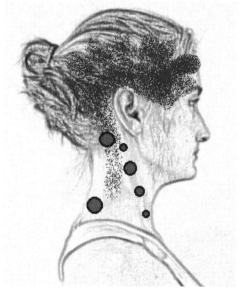

Figure 1-3

People often come to me thinking that they are having migraines because their headaches are so bad. They believe their migraine medication is not helping because it's not strong enough. So they take higher doses, but to no avail.

These patients don't think they are having tension headaches because they have been led to believe that tension headaches are moderate headaches. Migraine headaches, on the other hand, are labeled as severe headaches. Because the pain these patients feel from tension headaches is so crippling that it incapacitates them and affects their quality of life, they believe they must be having a migraine headache.

Tension headaches can be just as bad as, if not worse than, a migraine headache. The good news is that tension headaches are easier to treat with muscle therapy than migraines because they respond quickly to chiropractic care and massage therapy.

Migraine Headaches

People suffering from migraine headaches often describe their head pain as nauseating and usually report disturbances in their vision.

A migraine is characterized by severe pain in the head (usually on one side) that may trigger nausea. Migraines affect more than 10 percent of the population, and people who suffer 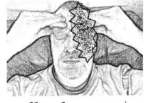 from migraine headaches can also suffer from tension headaches.

A migraine is caused by a change in brain chemistry that alters blood flow. Stress, a change in hormones, certain foods, alcohol, barometric pressure, and many other factors may affect brain chemistry. The chemical reaction causes the arteries to swell, resulting in the throbbing pain reported by migraine suffers; classic migraines are caused by inflammation of the temporal artery.

The pain of a migraine headache is usually one-sided, although a third of suffers have pain bilaterally. Attacks are extremely debilitating and cause neurological symptoms like dizziness, extreme sensitivity of the senses (sound, light, touch, taste, and smell), tingling or numbness in the face or extremities, visual disturbances, and nausea (sometimes to the point of vomiting). Migraine attacks can last as long as seventy-two hours or as short as four hours.

A classic migraine produces an aura twenty to sixty minutes before it strikes. During this time, a person may see flashes of light, dots, or wavy lines before the head pain sets in.

Migraines can follow hormonal cycles and may occur right before a woman's period when her estrogen levels drop. The hormones injected into our supply of meat also affect the body's levels of various hormones. For this reason, among many others, I advise everyone to eat hormone-free meat.

Food sensitivities and stress are other triggers of migraines because they too can change your biochemistry and increase inflammation in your system. Diet and lifestyle changes are required to treat migraine headaches and are discussed later in this book.

Cluster Headaches

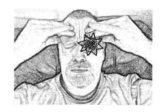

People who suffer from cluster headaches report their pain as in and around one eye.

Cluster headaches are not as common as other types of headaches. Fewer than 0.2 percent of people suffer from this type of head pain. Cluster headaches are severe, intense headaches that are short in duration, but they happen one to three times a day for a period of time—normally a couple of months. Cluster headaches also usually occur around the same time of year.

Cluster headaches are linked to the body's circadian rhythm (internal biological clock). The link between cluster headaches and the internal clock isn't fully understood. One theory is that the trigeminal nerve, the main sensory nerve of the face, has a relationship with the "clock" in the hypothalamus in your brain.

The trigeminal nerve exits the brain and sends signals to the face. It also performs automatic responses, like eyes when your eyes tear up. There is one for each side of your face.

The internal clock and the trigeminal nerve communicate with one another. So if the trigeminal nerve is vulnerable and receives a signal from the internal clock, that signal can be the last straw that causes the trigeminal nerve to escalate into an inflamed state, which then elicits the classic eye pain.

Usually just one side is triggered, causing pain that radiates into the eye on that side. It is worse than sciatica because the trigeminal nerve is a cranial nerve, closely linked to the brain. So when it screams, "Face pain," it is heard all too well by the brain. Unfortunately, the pain is usually worse at night, which affects sleep. Remember, sleep deprivation can lead to other types of headaches.

Cluster headaches may stop occurring for months or years, only to return without warning. Like migraines, these severe headaches can respond to the lifestyle changes mentioned later in this book.

Chronic Daily Headaches

Chronic daily headaches can be a sign you're suffering from multiple types of headaches, each with a different cause. Eliminating these types of headaches takes major lifestyle changes and multiple types of treatments.

First, you need to identify the types of headaches from which you suffer; second, you need to determine the correct treatments to reduce the frequency, intensity, and duration of your headaches. Ideally, these lifestyle changes and treatments result in minimal to no headaches.

Any type of chronic pain, such as chronic headaches, can lead to depression and cause sleep disturbances. Make sure you put together a trusted team of healers (for both your physical and mental health) if you suffer from chronic daily headaches.

Often after a trauma, the healing process continues indefinitely. I have had patients who suffered from daily headaches after experiencing a head trauma, concussion, or whiplash.

I have also had patients who suffered from chronic daily headaches after having an epidural. Spinal headaches occur with a decrease in cerebrospinal fluid (CSF). A drop in CSF can occur with trauma, such as a puncture wound from a spinal tap or an epidural. If the CSF continues to leak from the puncture wound, it leads to chronic head pain for an indefinite period.[1] I discourage pregnant women from getting epidurals because one of the risk factors is having headaches for the rest of their lives.

Imaging and lab tests often fail to identify a cause for the pain of headache sufferers because they don't show how the cranium is functioning. This is why you must pay attention to what your body tells you, such as where the pain is localized and whether it is dull or sharp. By doing so, you can work with your preferred healer to develop a treatment plan for your head pain.

I have had multiple patients who have suffered for years with daily headaches, despite seeing several specialists and spending thousands of dollars. After making the changes mentioned in this book, they not only are freed from their suffering, but they feel better overall.

Secondary Headaches

A secondary headache is a symptom of a disease that is irritating the nerves and/or blood vessels of the head.

Sinus Headaches

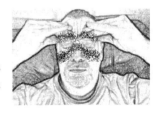

Sinus headaches are often described as having pain behind the frontal bones

---

[1] Fernández, *Headache: The Journal of Head and Face Pain.*

(the bones in your forehead) or cheekbones.

Inflammation of the sinuses can cause headaches, as in acute sinusitis. Allergies can also cause head pain. Generally, sinus pain is caused by pressure on the mucous membranes (the lining of the sinuses) because they are unable to drain well.

Mobilization of the skull (cranial) bones helps improve drainage of the sinuses. The skull is made of multiple flat bones that articulate with each other. There are no muscles that move these "joints," so they are considered "immovable." However, the flat bones of the skull are not fused together. A healthy skull has the ability to expand and contract to keep the pressure off the brain during changes of barometric pressure or sinus pressure. If the sinuses are filling up with fluid from sickness or allergies, the skull should expand with this pressure, allowing the sinuses to drain with this extra space. If restricted, the sinuses can't drain, pressure builds, and pain results in the form of a sinus headache.

Mobilizing the cranial bones allows for the expansion of the skull, allowing the drainage of the sinuses. This relieves the pressure on the mucous membranes, and the headache resolves.

Using a nasal irrigation system, like a Neti Pot™, may help as well. By cleaning out the nasal passageway, you rid the sinuses of the irritants that may be causing the swelling and remove the excess mucous that may be obstructing the drainage.

25

Head and Tooth Pain Caused by Jaw Tension

As illustrated in Figure 1-4, jaw tension can cause both tooth and head pain.

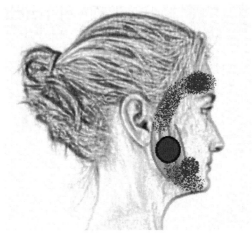

Figure 1-4

Temporomandibular joint (jaw) dysfunction can radiate pain into the head. Muscle tension in the jaw, face, neck, and upper back can cause pain in the head as well. I have many patients who come to me when they have tooth pain because it is often a result of their tight jaw muscles. If their tooth pain does not improve with their jaw treatment, then they see their dentist. If their tooth pain improves with their jaw treatment, they have saved themselves a trip to the dentist.

A bad tooth can also radiate pain into the head, making it feel like a headache rather than a bad tooth. Often such pain causes jaw tension, which can be misleading for health practitioners. They may diagnose a patient's head pain as jaw tension headaches, but the pain was actually coming from a diseased tooth.

With this misdiagnosis, the patient is prescribed an inappropriate treatment, so the condition worsens. Some patients suffer for months before finally going in for their dental checkup. When they find the root cause of their pain and their tooth condition is fixed, their headache resolves.

Medical Conditions Resulting in Secondary Headaches

Infection or inflammation of the brain or its arteries can cause head pain. Bleeding in the neck causes nerve pain in the head because the nerves that exit the upper neck supply the head. Arterial tears (carotid or vertebral dissections) can cause headaches, too.

Bleeding in the brain, as with a brain aneurysm or stroke, can cause head pain.

The brain itself does not have nerves for pain reception, but its lining and its blood vessels are very sensitive, so any increased pressure in the brain causes head pain.

Pseudotumor cerebri (an increase in pressure in the skull for no obvious reason) causes headaches as a result of the pressure increase.

A blood clot in a vein (unlike a stroke, which is a blood clot of in artery) can cause head pain because it causes the vein to swell, putting pressure on the brain.

A Chiari malformation can cause head pain, too. In such a malformation, the lower part of the brain falls into the spinal canal. As it falls, it puts pressure on the base of the brain.

This is another reason why, if your headaches are not resolving with treatments, or are worsening in anyway, an MRI may be indicated. An MRI can help determine the cause of your headache (or at least, rule out conditions like this). Such imaging can help the health care provider determine how your treatment should change, or if you need to be referred out to a different specialist.

Miscellaneous Conditions Resulting in Secondary Headaches

Extreme cold on the roof of the mouth (ice cream headache) causes vasoconstriction (the blood vessels tighten and get smaller). When the vessels re-dilate, you feel head pain.

Some medications can cause headaches, either directly or when their effect wears off. A headache that occurs when the medication wears off is called a "rebound headache." Sometimes the rebound headache is worse than the pain for which the medication was taken in the first place. This is why I discourage people from taking pain pills.

Dehydration is yet another cause of head pain. Liquids such as alcohol and coffee can cause dehydration and trigger headaches.

Liquids containing sulfates, as in red wine, can trigger headaches.

Coffee can trigger a headache when the effects of the caffeine wear off—these are called "caffeine withdrawal headaches." For these reasons, it's generally not a good idea to drink alcohol or caffeine if you suffer from headaches.

External pressure on the head (tight headgear or changes in barometric pressure) can cause head pain.

Other Headaches

Cough headaches suggest to me that there is a lack of movement of the cranial bones to offset the increase in pressure during a cough (Valsalva pressure).

When coughing, more blood is pushed into the head. If the skull bones do not expand with this increase of fluid, it puts pressure on the nerves and blood vessels that line the skull. Because nerves and blood vessels are sensitive to pressure, you feel pain at the slightest increase in pressure, especially if you are already on the verge of having a tension or migraine headache. The added pressure sends you over the edge.

Mobilization of the cranial bones often helps with headaches because it loosens the bones of the skull, allowing them to expand with the increase in blood flow. This expansion relieves pressure on the nerves and blood vessels that line the skull.

Exercise headaches and **sex headaches** suggest to me that blood pressure may be an issue. Again, mobilization of the cranial bones should help with this.

It takes a skilled practitioner to detect the subtle restrictions of the suture lines (the places where the flat bones of the skull meet). A restriction of the flat bones of the skull can cause an increased vulnerability to headaches. These types of headaches respond well to mobilization and chiropractic manipulation of the cranial bones, even years after sustaining the original injury.

There is a plethora of other causes of head pain. To name a few:

- Food and chemical sensitivities
- Vitamin and mineral deficiencies
- Exposure to certain mold in the home or workplace
- Carbon monoxide poisoning or other air quality issues

This is why you must have a good healthcare provider who can help you diagnose the actual cause of your headache.

Headaches are often difficult to treat because there is usually more than one culprit. You may be treating one cause, yet you may then get a headache resulting from something completely different. This complexity demonstrates why you need to have a team of healthcare professionals on your side, helping you get to the root cause of your head pain instead of masking symptoms with pain medication.

My Personal Thoughts on Headaches

I have read literature written by various medical doctors and neurosurgeons who have different opinions on the causes and treatments of headaches. Some even suggest all headaches are simply different expressions of a migraine, which is a swelling of the blood vessels of the brain caused by different triggers.

I believe they came to this conclusion because they see headache patients whose treatments failed them because they had migraine headaches that mimicked other types of headaches.

These patients likely were misdiagnosed because they did not have the classic migraine (in which the temporal artery is inflamed, causing one-sided head pain). Instead, the patients were misdiagnosed as having sinus, tension, or other types of headaches. Migraines can mimic these types of head pains if the inflammation is in a blood vessel other than the temporal artery.

This doesn't mean that there aren't other types of headaches. I personally have diagnosed a plethora of different headaches and have treated each according to the type of headache. I have successfully treated all but a few. The patients who continued to have headaches were not able or willing to make the lifestyle changes necessary to cure their headaches. Some patients just need to tweak their lifestyle, while others have to make major adjustments to their lifestyle as well as their career.

Regardless of the type of headache you suffer from, eating well, stretching well, exercising throughout the day, and sleeping well will cure you. Healthy habits help you deal with the daily stressors outside of your control, lessening the degree to which affect you.

But the question is, what eating habits, what stretches and exercises, and what amount of sleep will be best for your specific type of headache? I address all of these topics later in the book.

Chapter 2 : WHY DO WE GET HEADACHES?

ALTHOUGH HEADACHES may seem to occur at random, they usually are the result of a perfect storm of events where one is overloaded with personal triggers, to the point that they finally express as a headache.

The analogy I like to use is, "the straw that broke the camel's back." All it takes is a single straw to break a camel's back if it is already loaded to its max. Similarly, a minor headache trigger, like a change in barometric pressure (with weather change) can cause a major headache if you are already maxed out with all of the headache triggers you can tolerate.

This can make it difficult to determine your personal triggers. You may not even realize what your triggers are because you can normally handle the load.

But once you reach your threshold of how much you can

handle, all it takes is one more trigger, and bam, you have your headache. You may not blame that trigger because at other times, you may not have a headache with that very same trigger. The difference is that previously you were not as loaded with your other headache triggers.

Considering Headache Triggers

Many things influence whether you will suffer from a headache:

Genetic vulnerability: Some people are more vulnerable to suffering from headaches because of their genetic makeup. They may have hormone imbalances or just react more easily to what are usually minor headache triggers.

Going back to the camel analogy, your genetics determine what type of camel you are; your genes determine your strengths and weaknesses. Some are strong, long-haired camels that can handle colder weather, while others have two humps and can handle long periods of drought. Some have two humps and hair, while others only have one hump and short hair. If a camel finds itself in a different environment from what it has adapted to, it is going to suffer.

This is why everyone has different triggers for headaches and different degrees of vulnerability. Genetics partially explains why some people can drink red wine and not get a headache, while others will get a headache from just a sip of red wine. Or why some people can drink coffee and not worry about getting a withdrawal headache if they don't have their regular coffee the next day.

Some people have a trigger that is a big enough load all by itself to "break the camel's back" and cause a headache, while other people's triggers are like straws, and it takes a load of "straws" before they finally get a headache. Big logs are easy to determine and avoid. It's the straws that are harder to determine because they are only symptomatic when there are enough straws to finally cause a headache.

Overexposure to triggers: Eating the same foods, being exposed to molds, breathing polluted air, etc. can result in headaches. The load builds up over time until eventually it's large enough to cause a headache.

Poor sleeping habits: The brain needs rest to be well. It's easier to break a camel's back when it is tired.

General poor health: A compromised immune system makes you vulnerable to even your smallest headache triggers. Again, it is easier to break the back of a sick camel than a healthy camel.

Stress: Stress tenses muscles, which can trigger a headache. Long-term stress will compromise the body's immune system, leading to poor health and more vulnerability to even minor headache triggers.

So to prevent headaches, you need to do two things:

- Find out your triggers and minimize your exposure to them
- Keep your body healthy by sleeping well, eating well, and exercising and stretching well

You may not be able to avoid all of your triggers, but the more you control the ones you can, the less load you will have. Then when you have unavoidable loads you have to carry, you'll be able to tolerate them better.

Chapter 3 : WARNING SIGNS THAT YOUR HEADACHE IS A SIGN OF A SERIOUS CONDITION

BEFORE I REVEAL how to cure your headaches, first I must inform you when it is imperative to seek medical attention. It would be irresponsible of me to say you could self-treat when, in fact, your head pain is a symptom of an underlying disease that needs medical treatment, if not immediate care.

If you have a new type of headache, if the frequency is increasing, or if it is more intense than usual, resulting in fainting or vomiting, seek immediate medical attention! It could be a sign of a more serious condition.

Seek immediate medical attention if you have any of these symptoms:

1. A headache accompanied by confusion, blurry vision, changes in personality, difficulty speaking, weakness on one side of the body, loss of balance, numbness, or facial pain. Your symptoms may be those of a

stroke. The National Stroke Association suggests using the acronym **FAST** to determine whether you're having a stroke:

Face: Does it droop when you smile?

Arm: Does one arm drift downward if you try to raise both arms?

Speech: Does it sound slurred? (Stick your tongue out—is it straight?)

Time: You do not have much time if you have these signs. **Call 911!**

2. A headache with dizziness and facial pain. If you cannot touch your face because the pain is so severe, you could have giant cell arteritis (inflammation of the arteries of the face), which can lead to a stroke.

3. A headache that comes on suddenly. When you experience head pain with no warning, it could be bleeding in the brain. A severe case may include a loud sound, known as a thunderclap headache.

4. A headache with fever, loss of appetite, or unexplained weight loss. These could be signs of cancer.

5. A new or progressive headache if you are over the age of 50. This could be giant cell arteritis or a tumor.

6. A headache accompanied by a stiff neck, fever, and rash. This combination of symptoms could signal meningitis or an infection.

7. A headache accompanied by dizziness. If you do not know your blood pressure, or if you have high blood pressure and are on medication, a headache and dizziness could be signs of

your blood pressure increasing or getting out of control.

If you have any concerns about your head pain, ask a professional's advice. You may waste a bit of time and money if no serious issues are found, but the cost of ignoring your symptoms may be far worse because it may lead to an early death.

If you suffer from headaches and know you don't have an underlying health condition, seek the advice of a chiropractor. In my biased opinion, they are the best health practitioners to treat head pain because they have the best tools. More on this at the end of the book.

Chapter 4 : TO TAKE OR NOT TO TAKE PAIN PILLS?

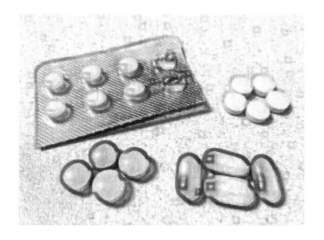

IF YOU TAKE PAIN PILLS for every headache and pain, this chapter is for you. I often hear from new patients that they take over-the-counter pain relievers almost every day for their headaches! After they learn to move their body more often throughout the day, eat healthier, avoid their personal triggers, and allow for more sleep, they often find they no longer need to take pain relievers.

Why an Easy Solution Can Be Harmful

When people have a headache, the first thing they usually reach for is an everyday painkiller like aspirin. However, nonsteroidal anti-inflammatory drugs (NSAIDs), like acetaminophen or aspirin, are not as safe to take as many people think. Such drugs have side effects and are very hard on the liver and kidneys, and can lead to organ failure and early death.

Indeed, I know people who take several OTC (over-the-counter) pain relievers every day and have for years. But some people get away with smoking for years, too, and never develop cancer or COPD (chronic obstructive pulmonary disease). This does not mean smoking is safe. In the same way, people who take pain relievers every day do so at a cost to their overall health.

Don't get me wrong. I'm grateful to have access to medicines; they definitely have their uses. But America has a problem with overprescribing drugs. As an example, 99 percent of the world's Vicodin is prescribed in the United States.[2]

I have treated many people who were taking so many medications that they had to keep a written list of them. Some of these drugs were prescribed to treat the side effects of the medications they were taking for their original complaint. Sadly, instead of curing their condition, the medications were muting the symptoms of their disease.

---

[2] "Nearly 100 Percent of the World's Vicodin Prescriptions Are Used in U.S." Vicodin Addiction. www.addictionvicodin.com/addiction-news/all-the-worlds-vicodin-prescriptions-in-united-states/

After educating these patients about lifestyle changes and herbal remedies, I helped them get off many of their medications (with their medical doctor's approval).

Medication is great for the short term because it offers a quick fix, but long-term use of chemicals is unhealthy. Prolonged use of medication leads to a decrease in quality of life. Such patients may be living with less pain, but at what cost to their body?

Consider this startling statistic: "NSAID use causes nearly 103,000 hospitalizations and 16,500 deaths. More people die each year from NSAIDs-related complications than from AIDS and cervical cancer in the US."[3] Furthermore, I have had too many patients in their late sixties find out that they have 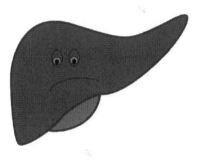 stage three kidney failure because of their NSAID usage over the years. And I have known of too many people who have died of liver failure because of acetaminophen usage.[4]

Why Avoiding Pain Relievers Is a Better Solution

So how do you balance the speed of pain relief that NSAIDs bring with their potential harmful effects? First, try other

---

[3] "Study Shows Long-term Use of NSAIDs Causes Severe Intestinal Damage." American Gastroenterological Association.

[4] Zimmerman, "Drugs Used to Treat Rheumatic and Musculospastic Disease."

treatments to relieve your discomfort. If you take pain pills every day, their effectiveness wears off over time, and eventually you will have a difficult time overcoming the pain, even with pain relievers.

Again, I do not believe in masking pain—we have pain for a reason. You do not want to turn off your body's alarm system. It would be like taking the battery out of the fire alarms in your home so you don't have to listen to them beep as your house burns down.

Once you start taking pain medication, your nerves are being unnaturally suppressed. They then become more sensitive to irritations that cause pain once that suppression wears off. As a result, you lose your ability to naturally deal with pain, and you become more dependent on pain pills.

If you are not suffering from a traumatic injury but from chronic aches and pains, finding the root source of the pain and treating it through diet, stretches, and exercises instead of masking the pain is far healthier in the long run.

If you are taking pain relievers regularly, *stop*!

The fast and easy path for relieving headaches is to take pain medication, but it is also the path to a shorter lifespan. If you take a pain pill for every headache, your body will adapt and be able to better process the pain medication, making it less effective for your pain. As a result, you will have to take stronger and stronger doses to achieve the same effect over time, harming your organs more and more until something fails and you become seriously ill and die before your time.

Yes, you will feel *awful* for a few weeks as you find other ways to treat your headaches, but tough it out. Once your body re-acclimates to a healthier lifestyle, you will rarely be in pain, and even if you are in pain, you may not need pain relievers to alleviate it.

Chapter 5 : ALTERNATIVES TO USING BOTOX FOR HEADACHES

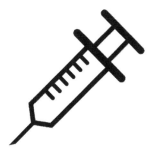

S OME PEOPLE USE Botox injections to treat their headaches. But if Botox can help your head pain, so can massage, chiropractic, and relaxation.

Botox involves injecting a nerve toxin into your head and neck. Researchers believe that this toxin alleviates headaches by relaxing the muscles in the face and neck. Self-massage, chiropractic, acupuncture, and other natural remedies achieve the same result.

I understand a patient feeling desperate and being willing to try anything to escape debilitating head pain, but relaxing your muscles by poisoning your nerves doesn't sound like a good solution to me. (And, I might add, that Botox injections are expensive.)

Instead, I would urge someone considering this treatment to learn self-relaxation techniques to ease their muscle tension safely. These methods should be just as effective (if not more so) without the cost to your health or wallet.

My favorite saying is "An ounce of prevention is worth a pound of cure." Before going to extreme treatments like injections of toxic substances, try the simple self-massage techniques, stretches, and healthy habits I include later in the book. Over time, they should help with your headaches.

Chapter 6 : ANATOMY YOU SHOULD KNOW IF YOU SUFFER FROM HEADACHES

LET'S LOOK AT SOME BASIC MUSCLE ANATOMY you should know if you suffer from headaches. The muscles I include in this chapter tend to have trigger points that can cause head pain. (Trigger points are muscle spasms that put pressure on a nerve and inhibit blood flow and lymphatic drainage, which leads to pain in another area of the body.) What follows are very basic explanations of where the muscles are and how the pain in the headache-inducing trigger points is caused. If you want more-detailed pictures of muscles, google the muscle names.

The Suboccipital Triangle Muscle

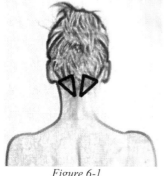

The suboccipital triangle (Figure 6-1) is made up of tiny muscles that help keep the head level with the horizon as the body moves.

If you are constantly looking down with your chin out, these

Figure 6-1

49

muscles strain to hold your head still. Chronic contraction of any muscle leads to a reduction in the flow of nutrients in and waste out, which causes metabolic waste to build up. This buildup irritates the nerves, leading to the sensation of pain, which sends aberrant signals back to the muscles to contract, resulting in trigger points. Trigger points in these little muscles can result in major tension headaches.

The Trapezius Muscle

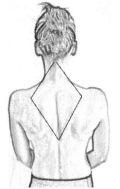

The upper half of the trapezius is the muscle that is alluded to in the phrase, "Holding the weight of the world on your shoulders."

Stress usually causes your upper trapezius (Figure 6-2) to contract with tension. This results in your shoulders tightening and rising toward your ears.

Figure 6-2

Again, chronic contraction of any muscle slows the flow of blood in and the drainage of waste out. Over time, waste builds up, leading to pain in the trigger points. Trigger points in the trapezius muscle can cause headaches.

The Levator Scapulae Muscle

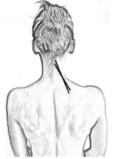

The levator scapulae (Figure 6-3) is another muscle that contracts when the shoulders raise up to the ears.

This muscle is under the larger trapezius muscle. It anchors onto the upper cervical

50

spine and inserts into the upper corner of the shoulder blade. Trigger points in this muscle also can cause headaches.

The Sternocleidomastoid Muscle

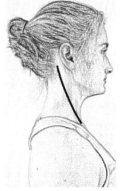

The sternocleidomastoid (SCM; Figure 6-4) is the ropey muscle you should be able to see in the front of your neck.

Trigger points in this muscle can lead to pain in the jaw, head, and neck.

Figure 6-4

The Anterior Scalene Muscles

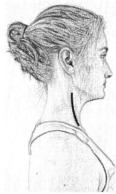

The anterior scalene muscles (Figure 6-5) anchor onto the neck and lift up the upper ribs.

If you tend to breathe with your upper chest, you can strain these muscles, causing them to get overly tense and leading to pain in the trigger points that can cause headaches.

Figure 6-5

The Temporalis Muscle

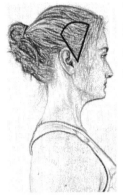

The temporalis muscles are the ones involved with chewing. If you chew gum or chew on chewy foods, you may irritate this muscle, resulting in head pain.

Figure 6-6

The Masseter Muscle

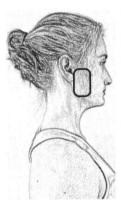

The masseter muscles are also chewing muscles. If you are stressed, you may find yourself clenching or grinding your teeth, not only irritating your jaw muscles, but harming your teeth. This can also result in TMD (jaw dysfunction and pain).

Figure 6-7

Chapter 7 : HOW TO TREAT FOR TRIGGER AND PRESSURE POINTS IN THE NECK AND UPPER BACK

P RESSURE POINTS are points on the body that you press to relieve a symptom. Trigger points are tender muscle spasms that can put pressure on a nerve, leading to pain in another area of the body.

In this chapter, I show trigger points and pressure points you can work on to see if it helps your head pain.

Trigger Points in Your Neck and Shoulders

You may find tender, bumpy spots at the base of your skull (suboccipitals; Figure 7-1), along the ropey muscles in the front of your neck (SCM, anterior scalenes; Figure 7-1), or along the posterior neck muscles or the upper back (trapezius muscle and levator scapulae muscles; Figure 7-2). When you find one of these spots, lightly press on it to see if it increases your head pain. If pressing on the spot increases your head pain, it is likely the cause of your head pain.

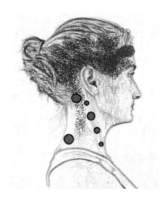

Figure 7-1: Trigger points in the SCM and trapezius muscles

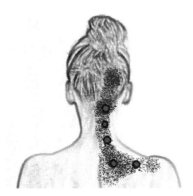

Figure 7-2: More trigger points in the trapezius and levator scapulae muscles

To treat these points, hold the pressure for three breaths. This helps squeeze out the metabolic waste trapped in the chronically contracted muscle. When you let go, new blood will flow into the muscle, bringing in nutrients and allowing the muscle to relax and take pressure off the nerve or blood vessels that are referring pain into your head.

If the muscle is still tight and sore, you can repeat this up to three times, several times a day.

You may experience immediate relief from your headache after working on such pressure points. Sometimes, it may take a couple of days before you notice the improvement.

Again, if your headache is not responding to your treatment, or if it is worsening in any way, see your healthcare provider.

Pressure Points Around the Eyes

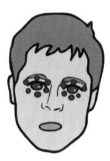

Figure 7-3: Common headache pressure points around the eye

You may find tender spots around the orbits of your eyes (Figure 7-3).

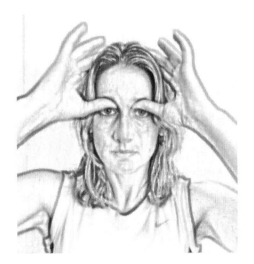

Figure 7-4 –Pressing on pressure points near the eyes

If you do, press on them for three breaths (Figure 7-4), giving yourself a type of acupressure treatment for head pain.

Pressure Points Along the Cheekbones

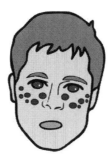

Figure 7-5: Common sinus pressure points

You may also find tender spots along your cheeks (Figure 7-5).

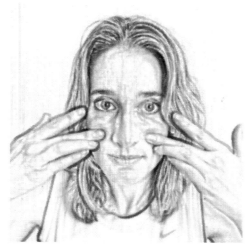

Figure 7-6

If you do, press on them for three breaths (Figure 7-6), giving yourself a type of acupressure treatment for head (sinus) pain. This also moves the cheekbones (zygomatic bone) away from the nasal bones just enough to allow the maxillary sinuses to drain.

Trigger Points in the Mouth and Jaw Muscles

You have muscles behind the jawbone that you can only touch by opening your mouth and sliding your finger behind the last of your molars until you feel soft tissue. These are the pterygoid muscles. They are very small, strong, and vital muscles.

Pterygoid muscles are used every time you talk, chew, and swallow (typically thousands of times a day). Combine this with the fact that these muscles are typically never touched, let alone massaged, and you can see why these muscles are very sensitive to touch. Usually massaging these muscles results in the trigger of the tear reflex.

Find a healthcare provider who is proficient in massaging pterygoid muscles to see if relaxing these muscles helps your headaches. If it does, have your healthcare provider show you how you can massage them yourself.

You can also massage the muscles on the outside of your jawbone (Figure 7-7) to see if it relieves your headache.

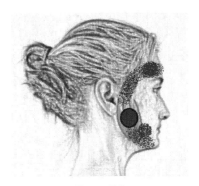

Figure 7-7

These muscles on the edge of your jaw are called the masseter muscles. Massaging these muscles can also help alleviate a headache. Try simply rubbing the meaty part of the jaw to see if it helps your head pain.

If you find any tender spots along your jawbone (Figure 7-8), see if pressing on them for three breaths helps ease your head pain.

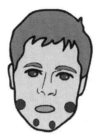

Figure 7-8

To see a demonstration of a self-massage technique to work on trigger and pressure points on the neck, face, and head, visit my YouTube channel:

www.youtube.com/watch?v=WTrduumit6U

Pressure Points in the Hand and Wrist

You can also try pressing on tender spots in your hands to see if it helps your head pain. The spots shown in Figure 7-9 are considered by many to be headache pressure points. At worst, pressing on these points will help your hands feel better.

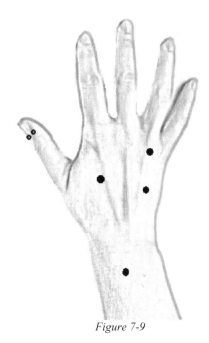

Figure 7-9

If any of these spots are tender, press and hold for three breaths, relax, and repeat up to three times. You can repeat every hour as needed.

If you find other tender spots in your hand, work on them as well. If a spot is tender, it's a sign that the tissue is not happy. Relieve the tenderness with the press-and-hold technique.

This helps get the fluids flowing in your tissues, thereby facilitating their healing. Treating these pressure points may also help your headache.

Other spots that may alleviate your headache are on the palm and wrist (Figure 7-10).

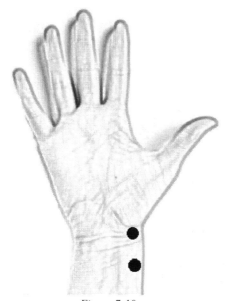

Figure 7-10

I find the most common tender spot for headache suffers is in the web of the hand (the thenar eminence) between your thumb and forefinger (Figure 7-11).

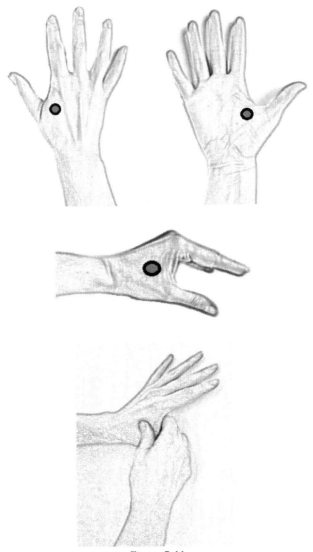

Figure 7-11

Pressure Points in the Foot

Other common tender spots for headache suffers are on and at the base of the big toes (Figure 7-12). If these spots are tender on you, try pressing on them for three slow breaths (breathing out twice as long as you breathe in), and see if they get less tender. You can perform three repetitions of this at a time, but leave at least an hour between treatments.

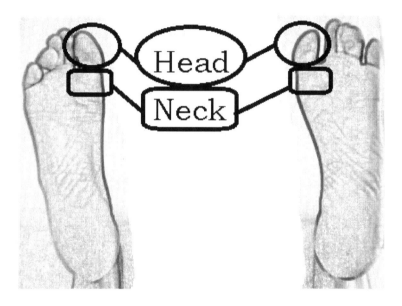

Figure 7-12

I have also found that releasing tension in the arch of the foot (Figure 7-13) often helps headache sufferers.

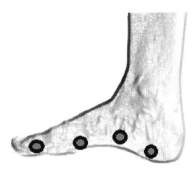

Figure 7-13

A foot massage also never hurts. If anything, it will help alleviate your headache in addition to making you generally feel better.

Pressure Points in the Lower Leg

This spot pictured in Figure 7-14 is the location of a headache pressure point in the lower leg.

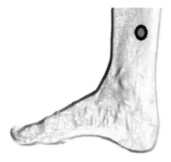

Figure 7-14

Look for points around your ankles that are tender. Tenderness indicates lymphatic blockage or muscle tension and tells you that something needs to be worked out. Applying pressure here could also be a potential alleviator of headaches.

Also try up higher on the leg. Feel the meaty part of the front lower leg, between the two long bones (the tibia and fibula; Figure 7-15), and see if you have tender spots there. If you do, press and hold for three breaths to see if this helps your headache.

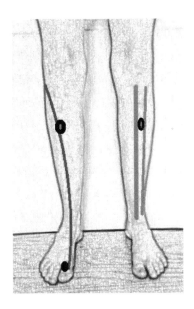

Figure 7-15

I find that it is better to do frequent, gentle cycles of pressure
point therapy than to do intense pressure a few times a week.
I teach my patients how to do the therapy themselves so their
symptoms do not return between their sessions with me.

Chapter 8 : CRANIAL MASSAGE TECHNIQUES FOR HEAD PAIN

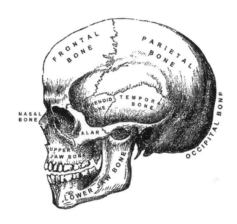

NOW LET'S LOOK AT how to mobilize the cranial bones to help alleviate any head pain that can be caused by rigidity of the suture lines of the skull. (Suture lines are the places where the bones of the skull meet.)

Temporal Press to Mobilize the Sphenoid Bone

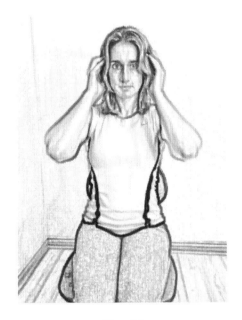

Figure 8-1

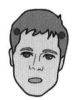 Bring your fingers to your temples (Figure 8-1) and press in with the right fingers, then press in with the left. This will wiggle the sphenoid bone (the bone outside of and behind your eyes) as well as release tension in the temporal muscle (which often helps tensions, sinus, and migraine headaches).

You can even try loosening the frontal bone (the bone that makes up your forehead) from the parietal bone (the bone that makes up the back of your skull) by pressing on the top of your head.

Cranial Mobilization: Temporal and Zygomatic Press

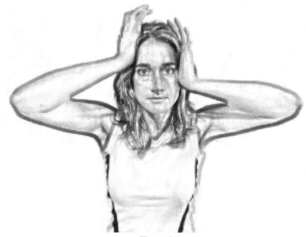

Figure 8-2

Place your right hand on the front right skull bone (the temporalis bone) and your left hand on your cheekbone (the zygomatic bone, also known as the malar bone; Figure 8-2). Then press your hands toward each other; your right hand presses up and in while your left hand presses down and in.

This mobilizes the bones that make up the front of your head (the zygomatic, maxillary, temporalis, and other skull bones). This technique often results in the drainage of maxillary and frontal sinuses.

Cranial Press to Mobilize the Occipital Bone

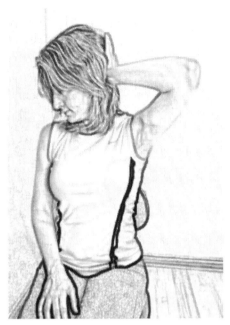

Figure 8-3

Place your left hand at the base of your skull on the left side, turn to the right, tuck your chin in, and press back with your head (Figure 8-3). Press forward and up with your left hand to really lengthen the back of your neck. Repeat on the other side.

Pressing against the back of your head not only stretches and strengthens the muscles in the back of your neck, but it also mobilizes the back skull bone (occipital bone).

This technique, when married with the temporal and zygomatic press (along with other cranial mobilization techniques), often helps relieve headaches (migraines specifically) induced by barometric pressure changes. A mobilized skull helps absorb the change of pressure, whereas a rigid skull results in the pressure change compressing the brain and its vessels.

(This cranial press is the same as the strong neck stretch in Chapter 9.)

Chapter 9 : STRETCHES AND EXERCISES TO REDUCE HEAD PAIN

NOW LET'S LOOK AT WAYS to loosen up the muscles that tend to cause headaches when they go into spasm.

For these stretches to work for you, you must do them often. It doesn't matter how intensely you do the stretches or how long you hold the stretches. *Frequency* is paramount.

If you spend an hour a day stretching, all it takes is another hour of not moving enough for the benefit of the stretching to be reversed. I advise doing two to three of the stretches in this chapter every twenty minutes.

These stretches don't take that long to do (some only a few seconds). The point is to break the cycle of immobility and compression of sitting over time. Unless otherwise noted, you can do these stretches either sitting or standing. If you sit at a desk all day, I encourage you to stand up when stretching.

As with any new exercise routine, confirm with your

healthcare provider that these stretches are appropriate for you.

Neck Rotation and Flexion

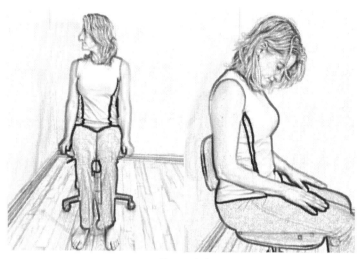

Figure 9-1

Simply moving your head left, right, and down (Figure 9-1) will stretch the muscles of your neck and upper back. These movements don't take long and are easy to sneak in throughout the day.

To perform the neck rotation, turn your head to the right until it's in line with your shoulder. Hold the position. Then repeat on the left.

When you look down during the neck flexion stretch, tuck your chin in. People tend to sit with their chins jutted out, which elongates and weakens the muscles in the front of the neck. Tucking your chin in adds to the stretch in the muscles in the back of your neck and strengthens the muscles in the front of your neck.

Neck Lateral Flexion

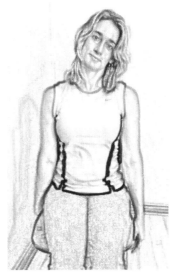

Figure 9-2

When you perform the neck lateral flexion stretch, you stretch the muscles in the sides of your neck. To do this stretch, hold your chair seat with your right hand to anchor your right shoulder down as you tilt your head to the left (Figure 9-2). You can lean your head slightly forward and back to stretch different muscles in the side of your neck. Hold each position for at least three breaths. Repeat on the other side.

If you are standing, hold your right hand with your left to anchor your right shoulder down as you tilt your head to the left. Again, you can lean your head slightly forward and back to stretch different muscles in your neck. Hold each position for at least three breaths. Repeat on the other side.

Neck Post-Isometric Stretch

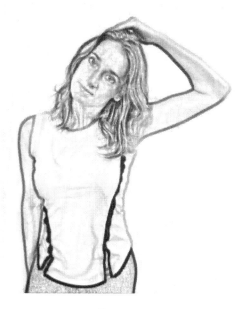

Figure 9-3

To deepen the stretch in your lateral flexions, you can perform post-isometric exercises that will release tension in your neck as well as improve the range of motion. For this stretch, place the fingertips of your left hand on the top of the right side of your head, and push your head to the right into your fingers (Figure 9-3). Using your fingers as resistance, don't allow your head to move. This will activate the right trapezius muscle.

Be careful not to push too hard with your head. The goal is to activate your neck muscles, not strain them.

Keep your shoulders down and away from your ears by holding onto your chair with your right hand.

Hold this position for three breathes and then relax your neck. After a muscle contracts, it relaxes and then elongates, allowing you to stretch it farther during the next stretch in the same direction.

After you relax, allow your head to tilt farther to the left. Do not force this motion. Once you reach your new limit, put your fingers on the top right side of your head again and press into them.

Repeat this press-and-hold stretch up to three times, then repeat on the other side.

Check out my YouTube channel for a demonstration of this stretch: http://youtu.be/PDcFpJuEoTg

Isometric Rotation

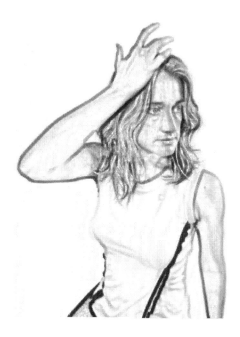

Figure 9-4

Isometric exercises require your muscles to work against resistance as they contract. To do an isometric rotation stretch, turn your head to the left and place your right hand on the right side of your head (Figure 9-4). Press into your right hand as if you are attempting to turn your head to the right. Don't allow your head to move; provide resistance with your right hand.

Hold this contraction for three breaths and then relax. You should be able to turn your head farther to the left with the elongation of your neck muscles. Again, do not force this movement.

Once you reach your new limit to your range of motion, press into your right hand again.

Repeat this press-and-hold stretch up to three times and then repeat on the other side.

Check out my YouTube channel for a demonstration of this stretch: http://youtu.be/PDcFpJuEoTg

Anterior Neck Exercises for Strength

To strengthen the muscles in the front of your neck, put your hands on your forehead (Figure 9-5). Press into your hands with your anterior neck muscles. Hold for three breaths.

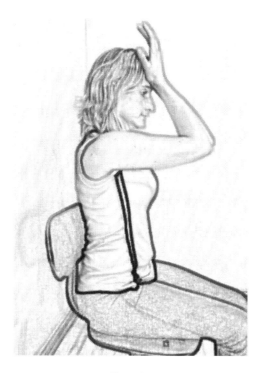

Figure 9-5

Lateral Flexion Neck Exercises for Strength

To strengthen the lateral flexion muscles, which allow you to turn your head, position your head so you are looking forward and put your right hand to the right side of your head (Figure 9-6). Press into it by trying to turn your head to the right, but resist any movement with pressure from your hand. Hold for three breaths. Repeat on the left side.

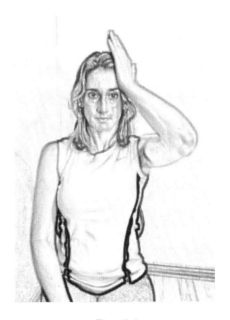

Figure 9-6

This stretch is the opposite of the isometric rotation stretch earlier in this chapter. In that stretch, you turn your head away from center and then press your head toward the center. In this stretch, you keep your head positioned at center and then try to turn it away from center.

Strong Posterior Neck Stretch/Exercise

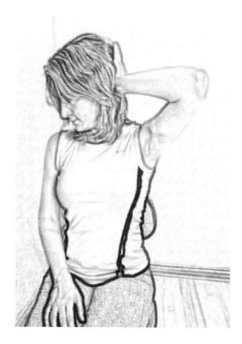

Figure 9-7

To work the muscles in the front and the back of your neck at the same time, try this exercise. Place your left hand behind the base of your skull on the left side, turn your head to the right, tuck your chin in, and press back with your head (Figure 9-7). Press forward and up with your left hand, providing resistance, to really lengthen the muscles in the back of your neck and strengthen the muscles in the front of your neck.

Repeat on the other side.

Shoulder Rolls

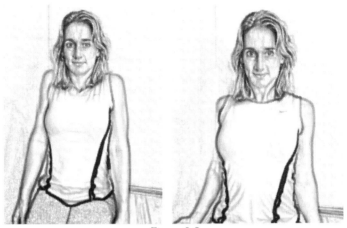

Figure 9-8

A good set of shoulder rolls can really loosen up your upper back and shoulder muscles. To do shoulder rolls, raise your shoulders to your ears and then roll them as far back as you can and as far down away from your ears as you can (Figure 9-8). Repeat this five times, nice and slow.

You can also do forward shoulder rolls; in which you simply reverse the direction. However, I do not recommend performing forward shoulder rolls because most people move their shoulders forward every day, and the exercise does not provide a significant benefit.

Breathe in as you raise your shoulders up, and breathe out as you roll them back and down. This way, you will marry stretching with a calming breath, which helps calm the mind (an important activity to do throughout the day).

Arms Over Head Stretch

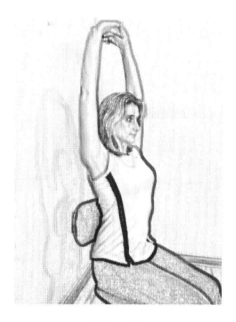

Figure 9-9

When you stretch your arms over your head, you work the muscles in your back and shoulders. To do this stretch, interlace your fingers and stretch your arms straight up over your head with your palms turned up (Figure 9-9). Keep your shoulders away from your ears and your elbows straight. Hold your arms above your head and breathe five slow breaths.

If you do this stretch while standing, be careful not to hyperextend your lower back. Hyperextension occurs when you stick your buttocks out too far, and this compresses the vertebrae in your lower spine.

Try it.

Sit down, and then stick your butt out. Can you feel how your lower back compresses?

Now reverse that action, tucking your tailbone in. Do you feel how your lower back stretches?

Now find the perfect in-between, where your buttocks are not too far back or forward. This is the neutral pelvis, where your lower back is in the safest position with plenty of space between the vertebrae of your lumbar spine.

Maintain the space between the vertebrae in your lower back by holding a natural stance as you raise your arms, which decompresses your lower back.

Shoulder External Rotation

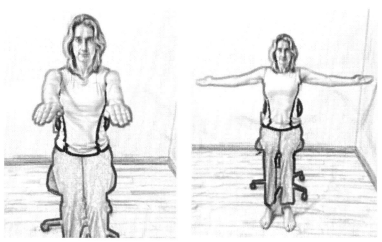

Figure 9-10

This exercise makes you move in ways you normally don't if you work at a desk all day. Stretch your arms out in front of you, palms down (Figure 9-10). Then bring your arms straight across the horizontal plane to the sides while turning your palms up. Be sure to engage the muscles between your shoulder blades as you bring your arms to your sides.

Return your arms back to the starting position and repeat a few times. This warms up your shoulders and works on external rotation.

Arm Raise

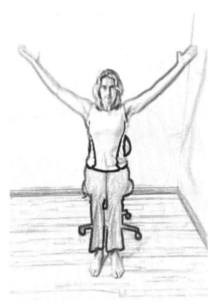

Figure 9-11

When you are at your computer for hours, your arms and palms are down the whole time unless you mindfully do a stretch like this. To do the arm raise, bring your arms up, palms up, to form a V, and squeeze your shoulders back and down (Figure 9-11). Slowly lower them back to your sides and repeat a few times.

It is good to do this stretch frequently. I like to do this one at least once an hour while at a computer.

Hands Behind Head Neck Traction

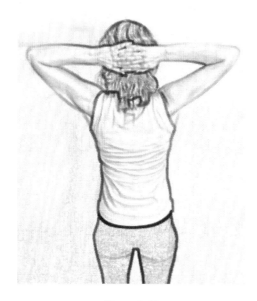

Figure 9-12

All day long, your arms are down in front of you. This stretch involves doing the opposite of what you do all day. Interlace your fingers and place your hands behind your head (Figure 9-12). Tuck your chin in, press your head back into your hands, and squeeze your shoulder blades together. Hold this for five breaths.

You can do this exercise either seated or standing. If you do it while standing, be careful not to arch your back too much; otherwise, you will hyperextend it (you want the mid-back to arch, not the lower back to compress).

Pectoral Stretch

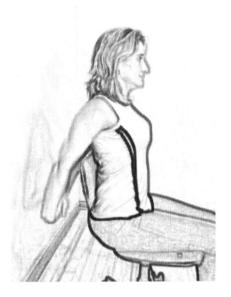

Figure 9-13

The pectorals are the muscles in the upper chest. If you work at a computer all day, your pectoral muscles get very little exercise. To stretch these muscles, place your hands behind your back and interlace your fingers (Figure 9-13). Straighten your elbows and lift your hands away from your buttocks (squeezing your shoulder blades together).

If you're doing this stretch while seated, arch your back over the back of the chair as you squeeze your shoulder blades together (your back may get a few pops in the mid-back region with this stretch). Hold for five deep, slow breaths and repeat.

A Standing Version of the Pectoral Stretch

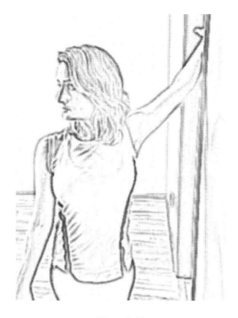

Figure 9-14

In this variation of the pectoral stretch, you stretch the pectoral muscles by standing in a doorway, placing your left arm against the doorframe at a 45-degree angle, and then leaning into the corner to open up the left chest. Hold for a few breaths. Repeat on the other side.

Arm-Across-Body Stretch

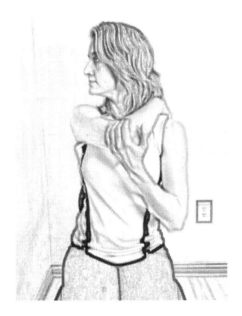

Figure 9-15

The arm-across-body stretch releases tension in the muscles in your upper back. To do this stretch, pull your right arm across your body with your left hand just above the right elbow (Figure 9-15). Do not pull too hard because you can overstretch the muscles. Rest your right hand behind your left shoulder. Repeat on the other side, alternating sides, up to three times.

You can add to this stretch by pressing your right elbow into your left hand, causing an isometric contraction of the muscles in the back of your upper right arm. Hold this contraction for three slow breaths, then relax your right arm and use your left hand to slowly bring your right arm deeper into the stretch.

Triceps and Lateral Body Stretch

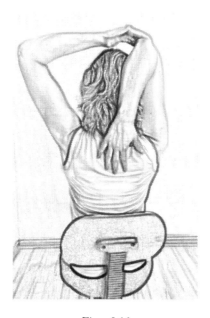

Figure 9-16

This one stretch works the muscles in the back of your arm and those down the side of your torso. To perform the triceps and lateral body stretch, take your right arm up, over, and behind your head, bending your elbow and hanging your hand behind you (Figure 9-16). Then use your left hand to pull your bent right elbow even farther behind your head. Hold for three breaths. Do not overstretch. If you feel a painful strain, then you are literally straining your muscles and/or spraining your shoulder, potentially causing damage.

Repeat on the other side.

This stretch is best done standing up, but it can also be done in a seated position.

Jaw Stretch

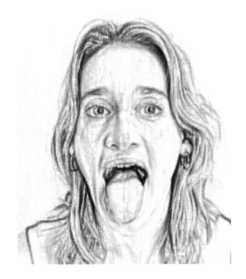

Figure 9-17

Your pterygoid muscles are on the inside your jaw bone, behind the back molars. These muscles are used every time you talk, chew or swallow, so they contract thousands of times a day. These muscles can get in a spastic state and form trigger points that can contribute to headaches. To relax the pterygoid muscles, stick your tongue out as far as you can. It also helps to make different facial expressions to exercise and stretch the muscles of the face.

Staring at a computer screen often results in a lack of facial movement, which contributes to muscle weakness and sagging of the face. That should be a motivating factor for some of us to diligently perform regular jaw stretches. This is a simple, yet powerful stretch. Try doing it every time you brush your teeth.

Post-Isometric Jaw Stretch

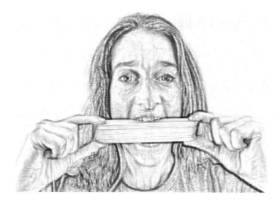

Figure 9-18

If you suffer from headaches and have a tight jaw, the tension in the muscles of your jaw may be a contributing factor. Your mouth should open enough to fit three or more of your fingers placed perpendicularly between your front teeth.

If your jaw doesn't open very wide, you can alleviate this tension by improving the range of motion of your jaw with post-isometric stretching:

First, open your mouth as wide as you can. Insert as many tongue depressors between your front teeth (as depicted in Figure 9-18).

Bite onto the tongue depressors for three breaths, then relax. Your jaw should open slightly during the relaxation of the jaw muscles. See if your mouth opens enough to squeeze in another tongue depressor. Do not force it, as you do not want to strain your jaw!

Even if you can't fit another tongue depressor in, bite onto the tongue depressors again for three breaths, then relax. See if you can fit another tongue depressor in or not. Then bite onto the tongue depressors for another three breaths.

Now that you have repeated this three times, hold your mouth wide open as you remove the tongue depressors.

Hold your mouth open for three breaths, relax, and allow your mouth to gently close.

This routine should help the range of motion of your jaw, allowing for a deeper stretch to the internal jaw muscles. Stretching your jaw every morning and evening until your range of motion is within normal limits should help your headaches. The question is, to what degree, as you may have other causes for your headaches.

Chapter 10 : A DIET TO DECREASE HEADACHE TRIGGERS

M ANY HEADACHES (and some types of dizziness) are triggered when you eat certain foods. In some cases, you may have a food sensitivity; in other situations, the headache may be triggered by chemicals added to food (preservatives, flavorings, etc.). You may also experience headaches because of seasonal allergies. Here is my dietary advice.

A Teaspoon of Honey a Day Keeps the Allergies Away

Allergies cause the sinuses to inflame, causing sinus headaches. If you suffer from seasonal allergies, try eating a teaspoon of local honey; the beehive should be within 25 miles of your home (as the crow flies). Honey from a hive close to your home is filled with the antigens of the pollen you are breathing in your area.

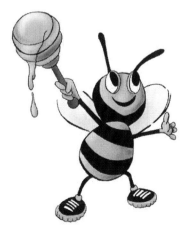

97

When you eat it, the body learns that the pollen antigens are "self"—something good that you assimilate into your body for energy—and not a "not self"—a foreign thing that needs to be attacked.

Honey works even better if you get honey made in the spring for your spring allergies and honey made in the fall for your fall allergies. Farmers markets are a good place to find locally produced honey.

Inoculation to Overcome Allergies

Another way to overcome allergies is through inoculation. Some people get allergy shots. You can treat an allergy by being exposed to a very small amount of what you are allergic to every week (but not enough to cause a reaction). Over time, the amount to which you are exposed is increased. Eventually, you are able to handle more of the allergen without a symptomatic response. I advise this be done under the guidance of a healthcare professional.

Eat a Variety of Foods

Food sensitivities are often the result of eating a limited variety of the same foods every day. This results in the body being underexposed to good antigens, which are the markers on organic material that our bodies use to determine if a substance is self or not self. Whenever the body is exposed to a new antigen, it attacks the new antigen like it's a virus or bad bacteria. This explains why unfamiliar pollen or foods can make you feel sick.

When your body is exposed to a variety of antigens, more antigens are marked as self and are not attacked. If you eat the same foods every day, not only do you limit your body's exposure to good antigens, but you make yourself more vulnerable to adverse reactions should you try something new.

The Rotation Diet: Keep Your Triggers from Accumulating and Turning into a Headache

For food sensitivities, consider the rotation diet. This diet will ensure that you get a variety of foods, and it will lessen your likelihood of developing food sensitivities, which is a growing problem in our culture.

The rule is simple: When you eat something, you can't eat it for four consecutive days afterward.

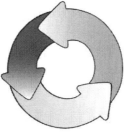

Think about that. How many times have you eaten the same food for weeks? How much variety do you really have in your diet? If you eat the same types of foods all the time, you will likely develop sensitivity to those foods.

Some studies suggest that you need to eat dozens of different types of vegetables to maintain a healthy gut flora, which is imperative to your overall good health.[5] The better your overall health, the more likely you can tolerate your triggers without getting a headache. So if you make a big meal, freeze the leftovers and only eat one serving of it no more than once a week.

Another thing I like about this diet is that after a week or so, you have to start hunting the vegetable aisle for something you haven't eaten in four days. Your veggies should expand from cucumbers, celery, carrots, broccoli, and cauliflower to include kale, leeks, radishes, spinach, water chestnuts, bok choy, Brussels sprouts, cabbage, red beets, squash, and more. The more varied your diet, the less likely you'll suffer from a nutrient deficiency—another potential trigger for headaches.

If you already have a food sensitivity, the rotation diet should help decrease your sensitivity to it. If you avoid foods you are sensitive to, you will become hypersensitive to them, and you may even develop a strong allergy to them. If you eat a small amount of something you are sensitive to and then avoid it for four days, your body has time to get it completely out of your system. Then when you eat a small amount of that food again, your body can tolerate it. Over time, your body should even be less sensitive to it. This process is similar to how an inoculation works.

---

[5] **A healthy gastrointestinal microbiome is dependent on dietary diversity.** Heiman ML1, Greenway FL2. Mol Metab. 2016 Mar 5;5(5):317-20

The Question of Eating Organic

When it comes to my vegetables, I am not too picky about them being organic because I feel that there is no such thing unless you grow veggies in your own garden and control how they are cultivated. Not all of us have that leisure, but if you do, eating fresh from the garden is the best way to get your vegetables.

However, when it comes to meat or any animal product (like milk or eggs), I am stricter. I try to avoid eating animal products that are not certified organic. Most meat sold at large chain grocery stores comes from an animal that has eaten who knows what foods, has been injected with who knows how many drugs and hormones, and has been subjected to potentially bad conditions that fill the animal's tissues with stress hormones. So I choose not to eat meat from those animals.

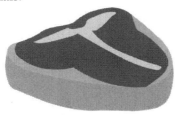

Hormones in Our Food Can Be Triggers for Headaches

If you suffer from headaches, especially migraine headaches, you may want to avoid meat that is not hormone free. Migraine headaches in particular are sensitive to hormone changes in the body. If you are eating meat unnaturally high in hormones, it likely will not help your situation. In fact, it may act as one of the triggers for your headache.

Where's the Beef?

I was a vegetarian for nine years but found it difficult with my active lifestyle to get the protein I needed. I had to eat more carbohydrates than my body needed to get the protein I required, and I had to take supplements for protein and iron, because I was borderline anemic. I was heavier then and not as healthy. I'm not saying it wasn't doable; it just wasn't easy for me.

I was taught that eating red meat increases cholesterol levels; all of my family members suffer from high cholesterol. But despite being vegetarian, my cholesterol was borderline high. I worried about how eating meat would affect my cholesterol levels. I found safe, clean sources of meat and even started raising my own chickens and cattle. Now that I am eating lean, clean meat, my cholesterol is lower than ever. I now believe that red meat is not the cause of high cholesterol. Instead, the overfed, hormone-injected, antibiotic-filled meat from stressed-out animals is the true cholesterol-raising culprit.

New studies also suggest simple carbohydrates cause high cholesterol. If your diet is deficient in cholesterol-producing foods, your body will converts simple carbohydrates to the cholesterol you need.[6] I was an example of this when I was eating more carbohydrates and minimal cholesterol.

---

[6] Boyles, "Low-Carb Diets Improve Cholesterol Long Term."

So don't be afraid of eating foods with cholesterol; instead, pay attention to the amount of foods you ingest that are high in simple carbohydrates.

When I do buy meat, I make sure it is organic and from cage-free animals. My favorite is from a local farmer who raises healthy buffalo. He even feeds them grasses from his own fields, making for very healthy and lean meat. I'm sure you can find a butcher shop that knows its meat sources and can vouch for the animals' living conditions, the quality of their food source, and that they are not injected with hormones.

Good Bugs Can Help

Another remedy you may want to try is taking probiotics. Good bacteria are essential to the well-being of your immune system. If you do not have good gastrointestinal flora health, your immune system will suffer, leading to immune issues like food sensitivities. Feed the flora in your gut with a variety of vegetables and grains to keep it healthy. As previously mentioned, some studies suggest that you need dozens of different types of vegetables to maintain a healthy gut flora.

If you take a probiotic supplement, make sure it contains more than one type of probiotic. You need a variety of good bugs in your digestive tract for it to be well. Many probiotic capsules contain only acidophilus because it is easily obtained from dairy products. This is not as therapeutic because acidophilus is the least deficient bug in our gut, especially if you eat dairy products like yogurt.

Additionally, purchase your probiotic from a reliable source. If you get it from a store, it may have gotten too hot or cold during transportation, rendering the probiotics useless (because they likely died in transport).

If you have to take an antibiotic, remember that it kills good bugs along with the bad. So take a probiotic during the antibiotic treatment and afterward to help replenish the good bacteria. Antibiotics make your gut vulnerable to a hostile takeover if not replenished with good bugs.

A lot of medical doctors say not to take probiotics while taking an antibiotic because the antibiotic will kill them. While it is true that antibiotics kill probiotics, I recommend replenishing the probiotics faster than the antibiotic can kill them. This way, the good bugs can overrun the bad bugs.

Digestive Enzymes

Food sensitivities may also suggest your digestive juices are weak. Ask your healthcare provider if taking a digestive enzyme daily with your heaviest meal is an appropriate treatment option.

Chapter 11 : ADDITIONAL DIETARY STEPS TO PREVENT HEADACHES

T HE FOLLOWING is my general advice on living well. The healthier you are, the less likely you will succumb to your headache triggers.

Drink Plenty of Water

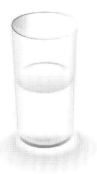

All tissues in our body need water. Dehydration affects blood pressure, muscle tension, and joint and fascia lubrication, all of which can lead to a headache. (Fascia is the lining that covers muscles and organs in your body, separating the different tissues while holding everything together.)

You can calculate how much water to drink by multiplying your body weight by 2/3 (0.66). The result is the number of ounces of water you should drink in a day. For example, I am close to 125 pounds, so I should drink approximately 83 ounces a day (125 x 2/3 = 82.5). Now, for every half hour you exercise, you should add at least 11 ounces. This is why I try to drink at least 96 ounces (three 32-ounce containers) of water a day.

If you drink black tea, coffee, and/or alcohol, you need to drink even more water. Tea, coffee, and alcohol are fluids that dehydrate you because they tamper with your anti-diuretic hormone (ADH).

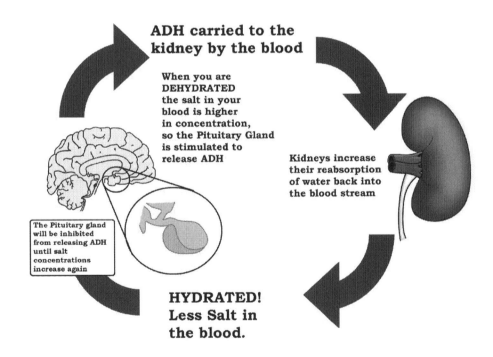

ADH carried to the kidney by the blood

When you are DEHYDRATED the salt in your blood is higher in concentration, so the Pituitary Gland is stimulated to release ADH

Kidneys increase their reabsorption of water back into the blood stream

The Pituitary gland will be inhibited from releasing ADH until salt concentrations increase again

HYDRATED! Less Salt in the blood.

Figure 11-1

The hypothalamus (a part of your brain) detects how much water is in the blood. If the water content is low, the blood has a higher salt content. The pituitary gland (the master gland of your body, also in the brain) senses this and releases ADH into the blood stream. When the ADH reaches the kidneys, ADH opens the kidneys tubules so more water is reabsorbed into your blood (instead of urinating it out; Figure 11-1).

After the water pressure goes back up, the hypothalamus detects this and tells the pituitary gland to stop producing ADH. The ADH in the blood levels drop, and the tubules in the kidneys will close down so more of the fluid will flow out into the urine. This negative feedback loop ensures that our blood holds the perfect amount of water.

If you drink too much water, the body has a means to urinate out the excess but keep a healthy amount in. As long as you urinate when needed, it is almost impossible to overdose on water, it's but easy to be deficient in water. So drink up!

When you drink tea, coffee, soda pop, or alcohol, ADH production goes down. This interferes with the regulation of water in the body, causing you to urinate out too much water. This leads to dehydration, which affects your health (especially over the long term). So for every ounce of alcohol and for every cup of tea or coffee you consume, you should drink at least 8 additional ounces of water.

Vitamins

Headaches may be a sign that you are deficient in a mineral or vitamin, like magnesium or vitamin B2 (riboflavin). Magnesium is a muscle relaxer, so a deficiency can lead to tension headaches. Vitamin B2 is important for nerve health. A deficiency in B2 can lead to nerve pain such as headaches.

There has been much debate over whether people should take vitamins. If you are eating a healthy, varied, and whole-foods diet, you should be able to get all of your needed vitamins through your food. Unfortunately, most of our food is grown on over farmed land, so the food produced on it is deficient of micronutrients and genetically designed to look good and have a longer shelf life (with no effect to its nutritional content or taste).

My general advice is to take a half dose of a multivitamin every day or two. That way you are less likely to be deficient in anything and you avoid the risk of overdosing on anything.

If you are taking a multivitamin, make sure the vitamins are coming from a plant source. Plants build vitamins via complex biochemical processes, producing one specific biomolecule. When vitamins are produced in a lab, an unnatural form can be produced and included in the multivitamin pill.

For example, vitamin E has two forms of isomers: an L-alpha-tocopherol and a D-alpha tocopherol. Isomers are chemicals that are the same but mirror images of each other. Sometimes this doesn't matter. For example, a cube is the same as its mirror image. But some shapes are such that the mirror image is different from the original. An example of this would be your hands. There is a left (L) and a right (D).

Vitamin E has a left and a right version. In Figure 11-2, notice how the carbon cyclohexane (the circle of dots on the far right side of the molecule) points forward on the D version and points back on the L version, just like if you held your hands with the thumb on the same side, one hand would be palm up and the other palm down.

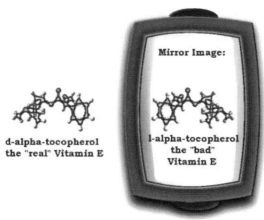

Figure 11-2

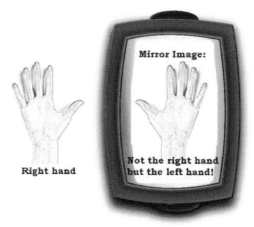

Figure 11-3

Do you see how the mirror image is not the same as the original item?

Only the right-hand version, D-alpha tocopherol, works in your body. To help you understand why one works and one doesn't, even though they look similar, think of a lock and key. If the key is just a little bit different, it won't work. Consider the example of a high-tech lock that is opened by your unique right hand. Let's say you can only open it by inserting your right hand palm down so it can read your fingerprints. Your left hand would not be able to open it. Even if your left hand had the exact same fingerprints as your right hand, it still wouldn't be able to open the lock because once inserted palm down the fingerprints would be in the wrong order and the thumb would be on the wrong side.

That's what happens with the left and right vitamin E. The right one works, but the left one doesn't. An easy way to remember this is "L is for liar."

Look at your vitamin labels. If it says the Vitamin E is dl-alpha-tocopherol, it has the unnatural form of Vitamin E as well as the natural version (hence the d and the l). In my opinion, you should throw this away because it may be harmful to your health. Look for a multivitamin that just has the d-alpha-tocopherol version of the Vitamin E instead.

Co-enzyme Q10

Co-enzyme Q10 helps with the health of the vascular system by decreasing blood pressure. If high blood pressure is a cause of your headaches, CoQ10 may help. If you are on medication, speak with your medical doctor before supplementing with CoQ10 because it often compounds the effect blood thinners or blood pressure medication.

Chapter 12 : FOODS TO AVOID

I F YOU SUFFER from headaches, you should know what substances are major triggers for head pains. By avoiding these, you may be able to tolerate more of the minor triggers. Here are some details on the major triggers.

Caffeine

Avoid caffeine (coffee, tea, chocolate, etc.) for two reasons. Not only does it lead to dehydration, which can cause headaches, but it can lead to a headache when the effect of the caffeine wears off.

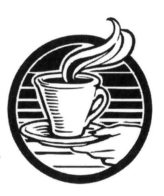

Alcohol

Avoid alcohol, especially red wine. Alcohol leads to dehydration (a headache trigger). Red wine not only contains alcohol, but it also contains sulfites, another headache trigger.

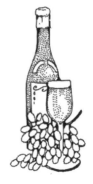

Soda Pop

Soda pop, like cigarette smoke, has many negative health effects. If you drink soda pop, try to stop drinking it for a month (including caffeine-free soda). The lack of caffeine can trigger a headache during the withdrawal, but soda itself can trigger headaches. Soda pop has a gross amount of chemicals, sugar, and salt. It ruins the taste of all other food and messes with your insulin levels, which causes sugar levels to go out of control and can trigger a headache.

Diet sodas are even worse because the artificial sweeteners mess with your brain chemistry even more than natural sugars do. Not only should a month of abstaining from soft drinks help to decrease your headaches, but it should also result in foods tasting better because your taste buds will no longer be overstimulated by chemicals.

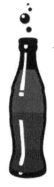

When you eliminate soda pop from your diet, you may find yourself eating healthier, and your body should show positive signs of this. I have had many patients lose dozens of pounds simply by no longer drinking soda and increasing their water intake. I always encourage my patients to stop drinking soda pop. To give them additional motivation, I tell them that soda pop has been linked to osteoporosis because it causes the kidneys to remove more calcium out of the blood. [7] [8]

---

[7] Mahmood M, Saleh A, Al-Alawi F, Ahmed F. Health effects of soda drinking in adolescent girls in the United Arab Emirates. J Crit Care. 2008 Sep;23(3):434-440. Doi:10.1016/j.jcrc.2008.06.006

Processed Food

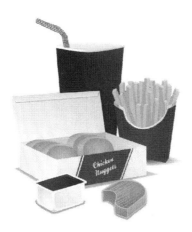

Try avoiding processed foods because they often contain triggers like preservatives (nitrates and nitrites) and flavor enhancers (MSG and aspartame).

Chewy Food

Avoid chewy food if your head pain stems from your jaws. Chewing on tough food can irritate the spastic jaw muscles. A major culprit is chewing gum. Avoid it! If you must chew gum to freshen your breath, chew for a few minutes and then spit it out. Chewing any longer than that risks irritating your mastication muscles, which in turn can trigger a headache.

---

[8] Tucker K, Morita K, Qiao N, Hanna M, Cupples A, Kiel D. Colas, but not other carbonated beverages, are associated with low bone mineral density in older women: The Framingham Osteoporosis Study. Am J Clin Nutr 2006;84:936-42.

Chapter 13 : IMPROVING AIR QUALITY

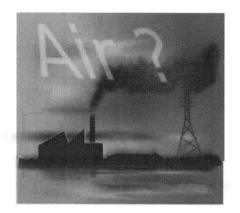

AIR QUALITY CAN CAUSE headaches. Air quality is mostly a product of your environment, be it in your home or office or the outdoors. Pollen, dust, pollutants, and other particles in the air can be triggers for your headaches. Some of this is out of your control, but there are things you can do that may help your headaches.

Indoor Air Quality

Dust, pet dander, and mold can reduce the air quality in your home. No matter how thoroughly or how often you clean, you can't eliminate everything that affects indoor air quality. Poor indoor air quality can lead to allergies, which often trigger headaches.

If you suffer from indoor allergies, think about getting better air filters for your furnace. I also advise putting air purifiers in your bedroom as well in your office. You should also clean out the air ducts in your home every year.

Using sheets and pillowcases that minimize dust mites and washing your sheets often will also help. In housekeeping, use high-quality filters in your vacuum cleaner and vacuum frequently. These steps go a long way toward improving your home's air quality.

Outdoor Air Pollutants

Vehicle exhaust contains multiple pollutants that can affect your brain chemistry and oxygen levels, so vehicle exhaust can be a headache trigger. Avoid your exposure to it as much as possible. For example, if you exercise outside, don't do it along a high-traffic road.

If you have a long commute, think about moving closer, changing jobs, or working from home more often. Not only is the air quality in traffic congestion unhealthy, but sitting for long periods of time is unhealthy too. In fact, prolonged sitting is now considered "the new smoking." You can check out my book *Top Seven Ways to Combat the Effects of Sitting* to learn more.

Cigarette Smoke

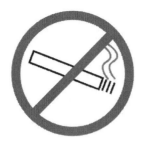

Avoid cigarette smoke, and if you smoke, quit! Cigarette smoke has a plethora of headache triggers. It contains toxic chemicals and affects blood vessels, including those in the brain. In this day and age, enough evidence exists about the hazards of smoking that it should prevent you from even picking up a cigarette. Those same facts should scare you enough to quit smoking.

There are many ways to quit smoking. There are patches, medications, and e-cigarettes. If these methods help you quit, then by all means, use them, with the understanding you are using them to help decrease your dependency on nicotine. If you are a headache sufferer, I would avoid nicotine, period.

Check for Mold

Have both your home and workplace checked for toxic mold. Every house has some mold in it, but if it is the toxic kind, it can cause respiratory problems and be a trigger for headaches. The spores in the mold can elicit an inflammatory response, resulting in headaches.

If you have toxic mold in your home, you must make sure it is properly, safely, and completely removed. This may involve tearing out drywall, replacing insulation, and more. For you do-it-yourselfers, this project is one that should be left to the professionals. Many companies specialize in mold removal. They have the elaborate gear to protect their workers from the mold during the removal process. As with choosing your healthcare professionals wisely, the same goes for the company you choose to check for and remove mold in your home and/or workplace. Make sure the company you choose uses products that are safe for humans. You may want to avoid the location until everything has aired out and is tested free of toxic mold.

Carbon Monoxide Detectors

You should have a carbon monoxide detector in your home. I have had a few patients whose headaches were caused by low doses of carbon monoxide in their home as a result of their furnace exhaust leaking.

Carbon monoxide is a toxic, invisible gas. If you breathe too much of it, your cells get deprived of oxygen, and your organs will shut down, leading to death. Early symptoms of carbon monoxide poisoning include headaches, dizziness, and shortness of breath.

You can buy carbon monoxide detectors at any home improvement store. If the detector ever goes off, call 911 and open a window to let in fresh air. Your local fire department will come and test for carbon monoxide levels and identify the source.

Chapter 14 : ADDING CARDIO WORKOUTS

WE TALKED ABOUT HOW movement is imperative to good health. When you move, your muscles stretch and change position more than when you sit at your desk or on the couch. These movements relieve tension that can lead to headaches. Exercise is also important. Boosting your heart rate for at least thirty minutes a day is essential for your overall good health (especially your heart). The healthier you are, the less vulnerable you will be to your headaches triggers.

Exercise

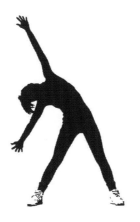

Even just twenty minutes of cardio a day will help keep headaches away. Find a physical activity you love to do because you will be more likely to keep doing it. Find a way to sneak in mini-workouts throughout the day. You will get more out of several five or ten-minute workouts throughout the day than you will with a one-hour workout every day or two. If you spread mini-workouts throughout the day, you keep your metabolism higher, and you should see positive signs of this, such as weight loss, fewer headaches, and a better mood.

Ways to Slip in a Workout

If you don't have time to go to a gym (or you simply don't enjoy going to a gym), find a way to sneak in exercise every day. The following are things I do to get a workout in throughout the day:

- I put a hang-on-the-door-frame pull-up bar in the doorway of my master bathroom. Every time I go to the bathroom, I do a couple of chin-ups and pull-ups.

- I do handstands throughout the day. Handstands are 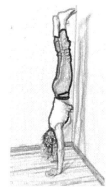 great for burning calories, increasing strength, and improving balance, even if you can only hold a handstand for a short time. If you can't do a handstand, do a plank or pushup. The trick is to do some weight-bearing exercises with your arms repeatedly throughout the day.

122

- o NOTE: During menses, I replace handstands with passive inversions, like laying on the floor with my legs resting up against the wall.

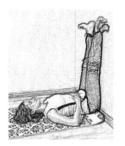

- I put a yoga mat in front of the TV so I can lay on it while I watch a movie and stretch or do crunches instead of slouching on the couch.

- During nice weather, I park my car at the far end of the parking lot or a block away from my destination. This easily adds a walk to my day.

- I take the stairs instead of the elevator.

- I find ways to stand up throughout my day. When you are on the phone, reading, or doing any activity you *can* do standing up, stand up and move around while doing the activity rather than sitting down.

- In the summer, I like to wake board. In the fall and spring, I like to trail run with friends (though they often get me to run in the heat of summer and the cold and snow of winter). In the winter, I go to an indoor rock-climbing facility. All year long, I love to go out salsa dancing.

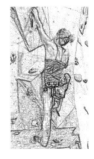

- Every year, I try to find a new physical activity to learn and try. I have taken karate lessons, horseback lessons, scuba diving lessons, and even belly dancing classes (to name a few). My husband and I have gone golfing, bowling, ice skating, and rollerblading 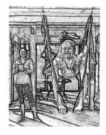 with our kids. This year, we tried the yoga trapeze (the kids love that one, too).

Find an activity you enjoy that involves some movement. It doesn't have to be an intense sport like tennis, basketball, or soccer. It could be something easier on the joints, like Pickleball.

Pickleball is a great alternative if your shoulders and knees are arthritic or too sore to allow you to play tennis. Pickleball is traditionally played on a badminton-sized court. The paddles used in Pickleball are made of wood or high-tech aerospace materials and are larger than a Ping-Pong paddle but smaller than a tennis racket. The ball used is similar to a Wiffle ball in that it is plastic and has holes in it, but it is slightly smaller than a Wiffle ball.

To play Pickleball, you serve the ball like you would in tennis, but the ball has to bounce once on each side of the court before the opposing player can return it. The first player to reach eleven points wins. The differences in equipment and rules, compared to tennis, allow Pickleball to be played by people of all ages and abilities.

Even bowling requires some movement and gets you off the

couch, no matter what the weather. Throwing a bowling ball down a lane gives your neck, shoulder, and back muscles a good workout.

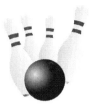

My point is, find activities you enjoy! The last thing you need is something else that feels like a job or a chore. Keep it fun, and you will look forward to doing your chosen exercise (or exercises). You will also be less likely to experience burnout.

Laugh

Laughter is good medicine. It releases endorphins that are natural pain reducers. To keep headaches away, laugh throughout the day. Laughter can also be great exercise; it gets the jaw muscles moving, releasing any chronic tension you may have in them. Remember, jaw tension can be a headache trigger. Bonus, laughing burns a surprising amount of calories

To get in your daily dose of laughter, listen to podcasts of comedians you enjoy, read a funny book, watch a comedy, tell jokes with your kids. The idea is to find ways to lighten up your day and laugh.

Life is short, and time goes by in a blink. So find ways to exercise that make you happy. Your happiness should be your number one priority. When you are happy, your happiness spreads to your loved ones. Similarly, being miserable is contagious. When you are miserable, you make those around you more miserable. This does no one any good.

Chapter 15 : PRACTICING GOOD SLEEP HABITS

SLEEP DEPRIVATION CAN BE a trigger for headaches. For optimal health, make sure to get at least eight hours of sleep every night. Studies have suggested that to be healthy, people should get seven to nine hours of sleep a night.

If you get less than six hours of sleep, you are at a high risk of cancer and early death from disease. Sleep deprivation also makes you vulnerable, and if you tend to get headaches, sleep deprivation will increase your vulnerability to your headache triggers.

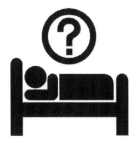

Research has found that the brain chemistry changes when

you are sleep deprived, making you vulnerable to pain. Sleep deprivation can also increase the frequency and intensity of headaches.[9]

Regulating Your Sleep Cycle

You have an internal clock that is regulated by the amount of light shining into your eyes. If there is a bright light overhead or shining into your eyes from a screen, your brain thinks it is high noon. This prevents the brain from producing the hormones necessary to prepare the body for sleep.

If you have trouble sleeping, there are plenty of simple lifestyle changes that can make a difference. One major change is to avoid overhead lighting and looking at backlit screens for at least two hours before going to bed. This lets your body know bedtime is approaching.

To mimic a sunset, use lamps set lower to the ground for a few hours before going to bed. If you must look at a screen, get red glasses because they block the blue light that halts the production of melatonin, which is needed for sleep. The reduction in blue light helps your brain's internal clock realize that it's no longer daytime and that it needs to release hormones (like melatonin) to prepare your body for sleep. Good sleep habits are imperative in combatting headaches.

I believe the two-sleep cycle is very normal, especially for people whose ancestry includes people who lived far from the

---

[9] "REM Sleep Deprivation Plays a Role in Chronic Migraine." American Headache Society.

equator. Before the advent of artificial light, people would go to bed when it got dark outside. In the winter, depending on where you lived, this could be as early as 5 p.m. Then you would wake up in the middle of the night, stoke the fire, have some fun, go back to bed, and sleep until the sun warmed up the day (8 a.m. or later).

In the summer when the days are longer, people wouldn't go to bed until late. They'd get up with the sunrise (5 a.m.) but then take a siesta in the middle of the day. Nowadays, we do not follow the natural rhythms, and our brains suffer because of it.

If you find yourself waking up in the middle of the night, let yourself enjoy that time with some light activity, then go back to sleep the moment you feel tired (no longer than two hours later). If you do this, let yourself have a nap sometime during the day. Don't force yourself awake, or try stimulants like caffeine because both are triggers for headaches. See if following your natural sleep pattern helps with your headaches.

Mattresses and Sleep Positions

For good quality sleep, I cannot stress the importance of having the best possible mattress. You (hopefully) sleep at least eight hours of every twenty-four hours. This is one-third of your life. If you are going to spend money on one item, it should be your mattress.

Your mattress should be firm for support with at least an inch of foam on top to minimize pressure on your body. I recommend a separate foam topper so you can replace it every three to five years (foam loses its supportive qualities within this time). You should also flip the mattress every three months or so, which extends the life of the mattress.

The best way to sleep is on your back with a small pillow contoured to support your neck and a wedge pillow under your knees. When your knees are bent, your back flattens out and is fully supported by the mattress.

Not only is sleeping on your back better for your neck and back, but it also keeps your face looking younger because it keeps you from rubbing the skin on your face against a pillowcase all night.

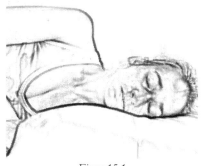

Figure 15-1

If you are a side sleeper, sleep with a thick neck pillow so your neck remains in a neutral position (Figure 15-1). If you sleep with your head tilted to one side, you will compress the nerves on the down side and pull on the nerves on the up side. The compression or stretching of the nerves can lead to headaches. You should also sleep with a pillow between your knees to keep your hips and thighs parallel to one another (helping to keep your lower half in a neutral position). Otherwise, you may be straining your pelvis, tailbone, hips, and/or knees as you sleep.

If you wake up with a headache or numbness in your arms or hands, you are pinching your nerves while you sleep, and you need to change something. If you wake up more sore than before you went to sleep, you probably need a new or better mattress. Talk to your healthcare providers and mattress stores to find someone who can help you with your specific needs.

If you still struggle with sleep deprivation, you may want to consider relaxation techniques and/or R.E.S.T., which are the topics of the next two chapters.

Chapter 16 : RELAXATION TECHNIQUES

S TRESS IS THE NUMBER ONE CAUSE of dis-ease, which leads to disease. Having a stress-induced headache is one example of a dis-eased state. To combat stress, you must learn to relax.

Relaxation is difficult in our culture for several reasons. First, we are all overstimulated! During our waking hours, we are bombarded with: unnatural light (which messes with our sleep cycle); unnatural sounds (which are amplified by speakers and earphones blasting straight into our eardrums); potent smells (such as perfumes, colognes, and deodorants); and expectations and demands at school or work. Every one of these is a potential trigger for headaches.

So how can we relax despite all of this?

Breathe

You have a huge diaphragm muscle that is designed to move with every breath. On average, you take 960 breaths an hour,

23,040 breaths a day, and 8,409,600 breaths a year. When you are stressed, you tend to breathe more shallowly with your accessory breathing muscles (like the anterior scalenes). These muscles were not designed to move with every breath. Your upper lungs are smaller than your lower lungs. If you only breathe into your upper lungs, you deprive yourself of the full amount of oxygen your body requires. Oxygen deprivation is another headache trigger.

This is why deep breathing is not only calming, but healthier. As you breathe fully into your lungs, you improve the oxygen and carbon dioxide transfer, which supplies your body with much-needed oxygen and rids it of toxic carbon dioxide.

Try taking a moment to focus on breathing out twice as long as you breathe in. If you can maintain this breathing pattern for more than five minutes, you should feel the tension melting away in your body. This technique is used in meditation practices. An added benefit of this breathing technique is that it increases the oxygen in your blood, which may help alleviate your headache.

Tense and Relax

If you are not relaxing with a breathing technique alone, focus on relaxing different body parts. Most people find it is easier to tense (or contract) a muscle than to relax it, so to relax your whole body, start by tensing your toes and then relaxing them.

I recommend doing this laying on your back so you can work toward relaxing all of your muscles. You can also do this seated or standing, but that limits how many muscles you can truly relax because some will have to remain contracted to hold you upright.

After contracting and relaxing your toes, move your attention up to the calf muscles. Tense them, then relax them. Move up to your thigh muscles. Contract the front thigh muscles, then relax them. Contract the back thigh muscles, then relax them. Move up to the pelvic bowl, do a kegel, and then relax. Move to the lower back, and contract and relax the lower back muscles.

Continue up the back, contracting and relaxing as you go. Move down the arms, all the way to the fingertips, contracting and relaxing the muscles as you go. Return to the shoulders, and contract and relax the individual muscles. Move up the neck, contract the muscles in the back of the neck, and relax. Contract the muscles in the front of the neck, and relax.

Contract and relax your facial muscles (smile and frown). Contract and relax your tongue (curl your tongue, stick it out), muscles of the jaw (open and close your mouth), and muscles of the eyes (look up, down, right and left). By the time you reach your forehead (raise and lower your eyebrows), your whole body should be relaxed.

The added benefit of this relaxation technique is that if your headache is from the tension in your neck, jaw, eyes, or any other muscle, contracting and relaxing your muscles will help alleviate your headache.

If you have a hard time relaxing with these techniques, you may want to try R.E.S.T., also known as floatation therapy and sensory deprivation therapy. I describe this in the next chapter.

Chapter 17 : R.E.S.T.: Restricted Environmental Stimulation Therapy

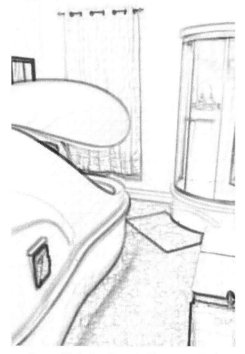

Figure 17-1: Dr. Karin's Floatation Pod

I HAVE A FLOATATION POD in my office for R.E.S.T. (Restricted Environmental Stimulation Therapy), also known as sensory deprivation therapy.

This is a great therapy to use to relax and de-stress. I got one mainly for myself, as stress is a cause of dis-ease, which leads to disease. Being a working mother, I have several stressors in my life.

I work hard and play hard, and floating is a great way to relieve muscle soreness and to promote relaxation. It was a bonus that I was able to provide my patients with a therapy that is just now becoming more common in America, especially because it helps a large array of ailments.

What Is a Floatation Pod?

A floatation pod (Figure 17-1) is a huge capsule that is sealed from light and sound to provide R.E.S.T. (Restricted Environmental Stimulation Therapy). It has 100 gallons of water saturated with 900 pounds of Epsom salts.

Many people take Epsom salt baths to help ease their muscle aches and pains. Can you imagine what 900 pounds of Epsom salts will do for your muscles?

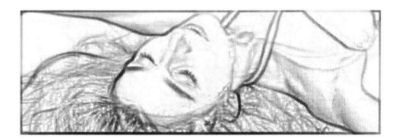

Not only that, but due to the concentration of the salt, you float effortlessly on the water. The body is less dense than this solution of water, so it floats like a cork does in water. This allows your muscles to relax from the inside out.

Once fully relaxed, you feel the space between your bones elongate and the pressure on nerves decrease. Your blood flow and lymph drainage also increase. The body is in a state that allows it to heal on a deeper level. Many people report that not only does their pain decrease, but that a sense of euphoria comes over them.

The Benefits of Floating

I got interested in floatation therapy because it is the most effective treatment for helping people relax, making it an effective treatment for all kinds of ailments, including headaches.

Sensory deprivation allows the brain to calm down, heal, and replenish, making it an effective treatment for those suffering post-concussion headaches.

In a floatation pod, breathing deepens, the heart rate slows, blood pressure decreases, stress hormone levels decrease, and a you experience a sense of euphoria and well-being. You become less sensitive to pain once you reach this state.

Brain Waves

There are different brain waves detectible by instrumentation (Figure 17-2):

Brain Waves:

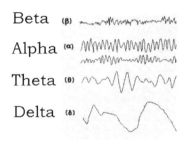

Beta (β)

Alpha (α)

Theta (θ)

Delta (δ)

Figure 17-2

1. The **beta brain wave** is associated with being aware, understanding, engaging, and actively thinking.

2. The **delta brain wave**, in contrast, is associated with sleeping.

3. The **alpha brain wave** is between the two; it represents a daydream-like state.

4. Then there is the elusive **theta brain wave** state. It is the state when the brain is "being"—when the person is not asleep, but not actively thinking or daydreaming either. This is the state that master gurus of meditation can attain despite external stimulation. This state is the most deficient in our culture.

Why Are Most of Us Deficient in Theta Waves?

Remember, we are all overstimulated! Most of us are overstimulated until the moment we finally crash from our awake (beta/alpha) state to our sleep (delta) state, skipping the healing theta brain wave state. Worse yet, we are rudely awakened by an irritating alarm sound, quickly transitioning from our delta (sleep) to beta (awake) state, again skipping the much needed healing theta brain wave state.

Feeling myself theta deprived, I bought a floatation pod to help me get into a theta brain wave state, to relax, and to help me tap into the brain's ability to facilitate healing.

Stress is the number one cause of disease (what I like to call *dis-ease*, because the body's state of unease makes it vulnerable to disease). So I value any way to decrease stress: meditating, exercising, laughing with friends, and now floatation therapy.

How Floatation Helps Head Pain

Remember, one of the causes of headaches is sleep deprivation. Sometimes headaches can affect sleep. This can lead to a vicious cycle. You can break this cycle by resting in a float pod.

One hour of floating is like several hours of sleeping. People who suffer from insomnia benefit from floating because they often can sleep in the pod. Many also report that they fall asleep more easily afterward and their quality of sleep improves.

Tension is another cause of headaches. Floating allows the muscles to relax because your body does not have work against gravity to keep you upright. The Epsom salt also aids in muscle relaxation.

Brain injury from concussions can lead to chronic headaches. The treatment for brain trauma is rest and avoiding stimulation like light, sound, smells, movement, etc. What better way to avoid stimulation than in a sensory deprivation pod?

Many of my patients report a significant reduction of their head pain with floatation. The only variables are the duration and degree of the relief.

If you want to learn more about floatation therapy, check out my website: www.orthofloat.com or the largest floatation center in the United States, located in Portland, Oregon: http://floathq.com/

Chapter 18 : GOOD POSTURE AND WORK ERGONOMICS

HOLDING YOURSELF FOR ANY LENGTH of time in an aberrant unhealthy position will negatively affect the health of your spine, cause neck strain, and may result in headaches.

Bad Posture Can Trigger a Headache

Your head is like a bowling ball sitting on a golf tee. If your head weren't permanently attached, it would fall off if not balanced on top of the neck. Similarly, if your head isn't centered on your body's plumb line (i.e., the spine), your neck muscles have to strain to hold it up. This can lead to tension headaches.

What causes your head not to be centered on the spine? Bad posture. Bad posture occurs when your head isn't properly aligned over your spine and hips when you walk or sit. Slouching is a big contributor to bad posture (Figure 18-1).

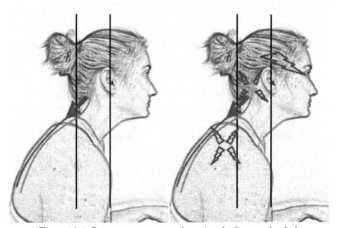

Figure 18-1: Poor posture causes neck tension, leading to a headache

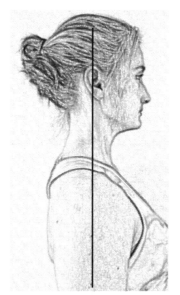

Figure 18-12: Good posture

Maintaining good posture is not limited to just sitting and standing. Holding items (even small ones) like smartphones, tablets, or laptops at chest level or in your lap causes you to look down for extended periods of time. This strains not only your neck, but your spine, shoulders, wrists, and more.

If you find yourself standing or sitting for a prolonged period of time, keep your spine in as neutral a position as possible. When using your smartphone, hold it such that your neck remains neutral (hold it higher than your shoulder). When working on your laptop, do not put it on your lap because this encourages poor posture.

To combat chronic strain, which can lead to headaches, move around as often as possible. It is important to move something every twenty minutes, no matter how proper your posture is. Movement gets the blood flowing, drains the lymph system, and breaks the cycle of extended muscle tension (a trigger for headaches).

Achieving Good Posture

Check your posture every hour (if not more frequently). I advise patients to do this by standing with their back to the wall, with their heels, buttocks, shoulders, and back of head touching the wall (Figure 18-3). This helps verify that their ears and shoulders are aligned with the plumb line.

People who are chronic slouchers often find this posture check difficult to do. If you don't make good posture a habit, then you lose the ability to sit and stand up straight. As a result, your health and appearance suffer; you will develop aches and pains, and you will have a hunched back and shoulders.

The good news is that if you practice good posture often, you will regain your ability to sit and stand up straight. (The older you are, the longer it takes, but it is still doable.) I can't tell you how many bent-over people who come to my office are able to improve over time.

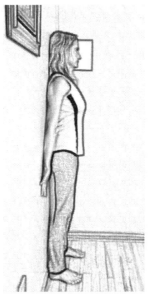

Figure 18-23: Checking your posture against a wall

Work Ergonomics

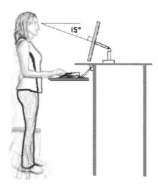

Figure 18-4: Proper ergonomics at a standing desk

More than half of my patients spend their days working at a desk. If it weren't for lunch and bathroom breaks, they'd never walk around. Research has proved that all of this sitting isn't good for us, but it's unavoidable for many people. If you spend hours and hours at a desk every day, here's what you can do to maintain good posture, reduce strain on your body, and make yourself comfortable.

The following is advisable for both seated and standing workstations:

1. Keep your chin tucked in and head back so your ears are over your shoulders. Jutting your head forward causes your chin to tilt up so you can see what is in front of you. This posture compresses the parts in the back of your neck, including the discs between your cervical vertebrae and the nerve rootlets that run

down your arms to your fingers; it also strains your posterior neck muscles. The farther your ears are in front of your plumb line (the center point of gravity), the more compression you cause. A severe slouch will compromise your whole spinal cord. Any type of pressure on your spinal cord is not good.

2. Position your monitor properly. Your eyes are "lazy" and like to tilt down about 15 degrees. If your monitor is too high, you will end up tilting your chin up so your eyes can tilt down. This too compresses the back of your neck. To combat this compression, bring your monitor to a level such that when you tilt it back 15 degrees, your eyes naturally look at the middle of the screen at a 90-degree angle. A good computer screen should be able to tilt and swivel. The surface should be reflection free.

3. Have a window to look out of periodically to exercise your eyes. If you do not have a window in your work space, find a distant object and focus on it for a few seconds every time you leave your workstation. I provide more details on this in the following chapter.

4. To ensure your wrist is in a neutral position, make 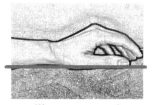 sure the bottom of your wrist is flat. The top of the hand will look like it is tilting up, but if you flatten the top part of your hand, you will compress the carpal tunnel, causing irritation of the median nerve, which can result in carpal tunnel syndrome (pain and numbness in the palmar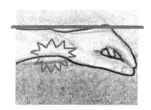

aspect of the wrist, thumb, and index and middle fingers).

5. Place your keyboard and mouse at the proper height. Your mouse and keyboard need to be at a height that allows your lower arms to be parallel to the floor. A good chair will have an adjustable height so you can make the adjustments needed for correct arm and leg positions. A good standing desk will have an adjustable height to allow for correct arm positioning.

6. Keep your upper arm vertical with your chest open and shoulders relaxed in a back and down position.

7. If you are standing, make sure your knees are soft and your feet are hip width apart. Wear comfortable shoes, and stand on a thick rubber mat.

The following are specific to seated workstations:

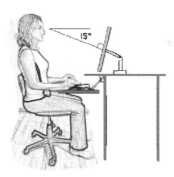

Figure 18-5

1. Place your seat should be at a level that allows your knees to bend at 90 degrees and your feet to rest flat on the floor. For those who wear high heels, this is a good time to take them off. (No one will see your feet under your desk.) This is a good time to stretch your

toes to help prevent bunions.

2. Make sure your lower back is supported by a lumbar support pad in the chair or a lumbar support pillow. A good chair will allow you to adjust the height and angle of the backrest to provide you with the proper support specific to your needs. If you keep a wallet or other items in your back pocket(s), make sure to take them out of your back pocket(s) because they will cause a pelvic tilt that can throw your whole spine out of alignment over time.

3. Use a chair with a solid base (a five-star base if it is mobile with wheels).

4. Make sure the floor is level and flat. I have had patients who had chronic back pain, only to find out their treatments were not lasting because the floor at their workstation was not level. They were holding their rolling chair in place all day. This strained their back muscles and constantly pulled their back out of alignment.

5. Do not sit cross-legged because it twists the pelvis, causing additional strain to the spine. It also compresses venous blood return, which potentially increases your risk of developing varicose veins.

6. Give your thighs room. Your desktop should be thin for maximum thigh space, with the keyboard in front of you.

7. Get up—preferably once an hour—and move around to get your blood flowing. Even if you just perform a mini-exercise, such as marching in place or doing some squats, any movement is good. It keeps you mentally fresher throughout the day, allowing you to work more effectively. This newfound efficiency will

easily compensate for the time it takes to perform such mini-exercises.

Chapter 19 : HOW TO PREVENT HEADACHES FROM EYESTRAIN

OUR MODERN LIFESTYLE , with its tablets, smartphones, and giant LED TVs, not only messes with our internal clock, affecting sleep, but it also causes eyestrain, another potential headache trigger. This chapter reveals how to avoid eyestrain and how to alleviate eyestrain if it occurs. I also offer tricks to help you maintain your circadian rhythm despite exposure to unnatural lighting.

Staring at a Screen Too Long Affects Eyesight

Have you ever known someone who took an office job and then had to buy stronger eyeglasses or start using "readers" or bifocals? When you stare for too long at any object that remains the same distance from your eyes, the small muscles in your eyes become fatigued, which can result in headaches and early deterioration of eyesight. This is why it is important to look out the window or focus on a distant object regularly throughout the day.

The lenses in our eyes are flexible, or elastic, changing as we focus on things at different distances from our eyes. Our eyes are better designed to focus on items that are far away than those that are nearby. (Evolutionarily, this was a result of having to be on the lookout for food, shelter, and predators.)

The eye is designed to conserve energy while focusing far away. Unlike most muscles that contract to work, the tiny muscles inside the eye (ciliary muscles) *relax* to pull their tendons tight. When we look at something far away, these ciliary muscles *relax* back into the eye, pulling the fibers attached to the lens taut, thereby flattening the lens, which bends light less so we can see farther (Figure 19-1).

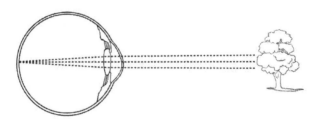

Figure 19-1: The eye (ciliary) muscles relaxing back deeper into the eye, pulling the fibers tight and flattening the lens to bend light less so we can see farther

To look at a nearby object, like a computer screen, the lens inside the eye has to round more to bend light more. The closer the object, the more the lens has to bend the light to keep it in focus. The ciliary muscles have to contract and move forward to slacken the fibers that normally hold the lens in a flattened state. Instead of relaxing, these little eye muscles must *contract* so you can see the screen, leading to eyestrain over time (Figure 19-2)!

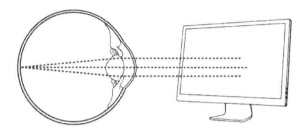

Figure 19-2: **The ciliary muscles contract forward to relax the pull on the lens, allowing it to round and bend light more so you can see things close to you**

As you age, the lens becomes less elastic; that is why most elderly people lose their ability to focus on things nearby. Now researchers are finding that people are also losing the ability to see far as a result of staring at computer screens for years. Again, if you don't use it, you lose it!

Tension in the Muscles around the Eye Can Cause Headaches

Muscles outside the eyes are responsible for moving the eyeball around. These muscles have to remain in their contracted state to hold the eyes still so you can focus on a spot on the screen.

Muscles were not designed to stay in a contracted state for hours at a time. They rely on movement to encourage fluid flow, bringing nutrients in and carrying waste away. Without this movement, the muscles strain as toxic metabolic waste pools around and within them, irritating the surrounding nerves. In this case, holding your eyes still to focus on a computer screen all day will cause head pain around or inside your eyes (another type of headache).

The Importance of Blinking

Another reason to look at distant objects throughout the day is that focusing on objects far away causes your eyelids to reflexively blink more frequently. When you look at something close, the natural blink rate slows down because you are concentrating intently on what you are looking at, and, however 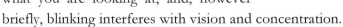 briefly, blinking interferes with vision and concentration.

Blinking helps distribute moisture over the eyes. Without frequent blinking, your eyes are at risk of drying out. Many people already suffer from drier eyes, often as a result of wearing contact lenses or having a condition like Sjorgen's syndrome. Staring at a screen, which reduces how often you blink, can make this much worse, even to the point of causing eye pain (yet another pain in the head).

So take time throughout the day to look out a window—or even better, go outside—and focus on objects at varied distances from you. Make a point to take a vision break every hour or so. Your eyes and brain will thank you in the long run!

Chapter 20 : FIGURING OUT YOUR PERSONAL TRIGGERS

KEEPING A LOG of your symptoms and lifestyle may help you figure out sensitivities and triggers for your headaches.

Writing down details about your lifestyle over the course of several weeks or months may help you discover a pattern to your headaches. Keeping a log will help you determine how important sleep, exercise, and quality of food are to keeping your headaches at bay.

When you see patterns, you can correct the behavior or avoid the trigger that leads to headaches. For example, if you get less than eight hours of sleep for a few days in a row, you get a headache later that week. Or if you eat chocolate, you consistently get a headache five days later. Or if you exercise daily, your headaches are less intense over all. After you understand the cause of your headaches, you can take the necessary steps to prevent them.

To keep a log, record your diet, activity, and exposures to potential triggers to determine the cause of your headaches. Figure 20-1 illustrates an example Headache Log.

Date	Hrs of sleep	Time of day	Food/ Drink	Physical activity	Headache Intensity & Duration
Jan. 1 *Put menstrual notes and sleep notes here		a.m.	Breakfast: Snacks: Drinks: *Exposure to any pollen or chemicals?*	*Any exercise or stretches?*	Intensity 0–10/10 Minutes/ hours long
		Noon	Lunch: Snacks: Drinks: *Exposure to any pollen or chemicals?*		Intensity 0–10/10 Minutes/ hours long
		p.m.	Dinner: Snacks: Drinks: *Exposure to any pollen or chemicals?*		Intensity 0–10/10 Minutes/ hours long

Figure 20-1

It may take months of logging in your dairy before you find your pattern. Headaches often do not occur until days after the exposure to the trigger, making it difficult to determine the original cause. But once you figure out the pattern, the rest of your life will be less painful, healthier, and likely longer. It is not the easy path, but it is the healthier path in the long run.

Personally, I (and many of my patients) have failed to keep a log for more than a couple weeks. As I was logging, I found I was living a healthier lifestyle, and I was less symptomatic because of it. I stopped logging but continued the healthier lifestyle, and I have been feeling good ever since. I am not perfect, but I have learned to cut back on how often I "cheat" so I never experience severe symptoms.

Chapter 21 : HERBAL REMEDIES AND THERAPEUTIC OILS FOR HEADACHES

YOU'VE TRIED ALL OF THE TECHNIQUES mentioned in this book to treat your head pain and relax, yet you still have a headache that you cannot get rid of. You'd really like to take a pain pill but know you shouldn't. Instead, try some herbal alternatives. This chapter lists the herbal remedies and therapeutic oils that I have found to be helpful. You can find these at most health food stores, but I recommend asking your healthcare provider what brand they prefer (quality of brands changes over time).

White Willow Bark for Pain

White willow bark is the natural version of aspirin. Pharmacological companies discovered the active ingredient in white willow bark that decreased pain, and now they chemically produce it in a concentrated form. If aspirin were developed today, it would be labeled as a prescription drug because its lethal dose is so minuscule.

White willow bark contains aspirin in its natural state and is less likely to irritate the stomach lining or cause death. It is more expensive than a bottle of aspirin, but if you adhere to the lifestyle changes this book suggests, you should not need much of this herbal remedy.

Valerian Root for Better Sleep

Valerian root is a natural sleep aid. If you have difficulty sleeping, which can negatively affect your headaches, valerian root may help. You can find it in pill form.

Kava Kava Root for Muscle Tension

Kava Kava root is a natural muscle relaxer. It may help take the edge off a tension headache.

Passion Flower for Relaxation (anti-stressor)

Passion flower can help you relax when you are feeling stressed or anxious. You can take it in the form of a tea, or for a stronger dose, you can take it as a tincture.

Caution!

As with any muscle relaxer or sleep aid, you should first try these remedies when you don't have to drive, work, or do anything that you would not do while impaired. It is best to take these herbs at night to help you relax and sleep.

Other Herbs That May Help

Other herbs that may help with your headaches are feverfew, black cohosh, and butterbur (to name a few). I would not advise using these herbs without guidance from a practitioner who is well versed in herbal remedies.

Therapeutic Oils That May Help

Essential Oil of Peppermint for Muscle Aches

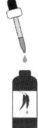

Essential oil of peppermint is good for tense muscles. It has a nice cooling effect, which also helps diminish aches in the muscle. Take three to four drops of peppermint oil and massage it into the neck.

Essential Oil of Clove for Muscle Tension

Essential oil of clove is also good for muscle tension. Clove has a nice warming effect, which helps relax tense muscles. Take three to four drops of clove oil and massage it into the neck and upper back.

Essential Oil of Lavender for Relaxation

Essential oil of lavender is a calming oil. Take three to four drops of lavender oil and massage it into the chest. Combine this with some deep-breathing techniques, and feel your stress melt away.

My Personal Advice on Using Natural Remedies

You can seek advice from a naturopath to find out if other herbal remedies would be better for your specific needs. However, like prescription medication, I am not a fan of relying on a surplus of pills, tinctures, etc. Natural or not, such treatments should be used sparingly so they work when you need them.

Chapter 22 : ICE OR HEAT THERAPY FOR HEADACHES

I F YOU ARE EXPERIENCING PAIN and are looking for an alternative to over-the-counter pain relievers, temperature therapy may be an option. Heat therapy and ice therapy are useful, and sometimes can be used interchangeably.

Heat Therapy

Heat is a great analgesic (pain reducer) and opens up capillary beds, bringing more blood to the region that is experiencing pain. This is great for tight muscles. However, heat therapy is also inflammatory. If your headache is caused by inflammation, as with migraines and other types of headaches, heat can make it worse.

Ice Therapy

Like heat, ice is a great analgesic. But ice is also an anti-inflammatory. Ice therapy is a suitable treatment for acute injuries (during the inflamed state) because ice therapy causes your blood vessels to constrict, which reduces blood supply to the region. But if you don't have any inflammation, ice therapy is unhealthy for tissues already starved for blood, as with tension headaches (which are caused by spastic muscles).

Careful!

Be careful with heat and ice. They are very effective tools when used correctly, but they can be dangerous when used incorrectly or to treat the wrong ailment.

Patients often make an emergency visit to my office after sleeping with a heating pad. This is a dangerous practice. It is too easy to overheat the region and wake up in a terribly inflamed state.

It is also dangerous to sleep with an ice pack, especially if you are on pain pills. I have had more than one patient wake up with frostbite under an ice pack after having slept with one.

The Safest Treatment for Headaches

I believe the safest self-treatment for most headaches is to

1. Heat the upper back (trapezius region) for ten minutes to bring nutrient-filled blood to the area and to relax the upper back and neck muscles.
2. Stretch the neck, shoulders, and upper back gently while the muscles are warm and pliable.
3. Finish with two minutes of ice to the temporal region of the head and the base of the skull to calm any inflammation that may have worsened with the heat.

Chapter 23 : DEVICES THAT MAY HELP WITH YOUR HEADACHES

T HE BEST TREATMENT for headaches is to avoid headache triggers because "an ounce of prevention is worth a pound of cure." But if you have a headache, the following devices may help you alleviate it so you do not have to resort to taking pain medications.

TENs Unit

A TENs unit is a portable device that can be worn all day and night to help reduce pain. It uses electrical stimulation to close the pain gates of nerves of spastic muscles.

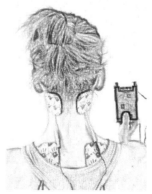

Figure 23-1

The device has four sticky pads attached to wires that you place around the affected area. Figure 23-1 illustrates placement of the pads for tension headaches: on the neck and at the base of the skull. You plug the wires into the TENs unit and increase the intensity of the electrical pulse until it scrambles the sensation of pain.

Once intense enough, you feel a massaging electrical current instead of your pain. This is a passive, palliative treatment, but there are no side effects (unlike pain medication). After the initial cost of the TENs unit, you just need to replace the batteries and the sticky pads (they lose their stick after multiple uses).

You should be able to purchase a TENs unit for under $100.

Effective Massage Tools

If you suffer from tension headaches, massage therapy is another treatment to consider. I prefer a professional massage from licensed massage therapists or healthcare providers like chiropractors and physical therapists.

Receiving a massage is better than self-massage because it is easier to get your muscles to relax when you're not activating your own muscles to massage them.

Having muscle work performed by healthcare providers, in my opinion, is even better than getting a massage from a massage therapist. Chiropractors and physical therapists have more knowledge of your condition, so they should be more effective at treating your condition.

Plus, they should have professional myofascial releasing tools like the T-bar, Graston instruments, and other powerful massage tools like the Thumper Maxi Pro Massager, the Jeanie Rub massager, and the RRT (Rapid Release Technology; Figure 23-2) to name a few.

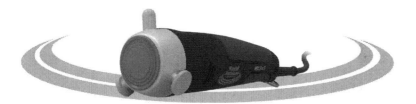

Figure 23-2: RRT (Rapid Release Technology)

I personally prefer using the RRT (also known as Rapid Release) because it uses painless, high-speed vibrations to melt scar tissue/adhesion versus the pounding action of slower devices or the scraping or striping action of contoured tools.

You can purchase the RRT online. I have had patients buy their own RRT so they could treat themselves more frequently in the comfort of their own home. The cost is high (about $1,500), but if you use the RRT thirty times, the cost comes to $50 per treatment. It more than pays for itself, as after which, each time you use it, the treatment is free.

You can check it out at:
https://rapidreleasetech.com/product/

Self-Massage Tools

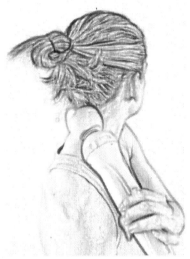

Figure 23-3

To increase the benefits of a professional massage, it helps to self-massage at home between your professional massages. Otherwise, after only a few days, your muscles may tense back up from your activities of daily living. If you massage your muscles daily, the benefits of the professional massage will last that much longer.

There are many devices at a wide range of price points to help you self-massage. I prefer vibrating massage tools with a long handle to make reaching the back of the neck and upper back easier.

Such tools run from as little as $30 to hundreds of dollars.

I also recommend tools like the Thera Cane and Body Back Buddy (Figure 23-4). They help you press on trigger points in the back of your torso and neck while keeping your arms down, which allows the upper back muscles to stay relaxed. The cost of each tool is about $40.

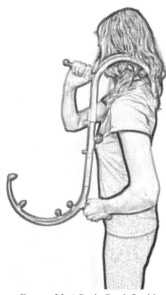

Figure 23-4 Body Back Buddy

Mouth Splint

If you have headaches from jaw dysfunction, talk to your dentist to see if wearing a splint at night is a good option for you. At a minimum, wearing a night splint will protect your teeth if you grind your teeth at night. Bonus if it helps your head pain.

Saunders Cervical Traction Unit

If your headaches are due to nerve irritation from herniation(s) in your neck, a home traction unit may be a good idea (Figure 23-5). Explore the possibility with your healthcare provider.

My favorite home traction unit for the neck is the Saunders Cervical Home Traction Units, as you can traction your neck at a specific poundage at an angle designed to open the space between the bones in your neck. It is very effective at decompressing cervical discs; so much so, many suppliers require a prescription from a health care provider.

You can find new units selling for less than $400 online.

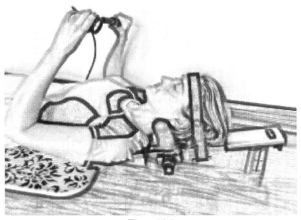

Figure 23-5

Chapter 24 : WHY SEE A CHIROPRACTOR FOR YOUR HEADACHES?

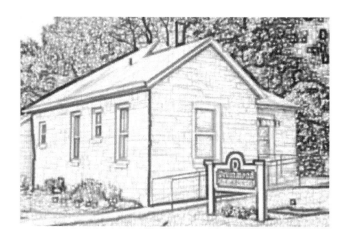

Figure 24-1: Dr. Karin's Office

S OME CONTEND THAT chiropractic medicine is less valid or less advanced than other forms of medicine. This is not true.[10] It is sad to me that many people still

---

[10] Bryans, et al., "Evidence-based Guidelines for the Chiropractic Treatment of Adults with Headache." *Journal of Manipulative and Physiological Therapeutics.*
Astin and Ernst, "The Effectiveness of Spinal Manipulation for the

consider chiropractic an "alternative" medicine or think that chiropractors just treat neck or back pain.

Chiropractors are primary care physicians who have as many years of education as a medical doctor. It only takes months to learn how to adjust, but years to learn differential diagnosis. A chiropractor knows when not to manipulate, when to refer a patient to someone else, and which specialist the patient should be referred to, if need be.

There is little mystery on why chiropractic works. It has been scientifically studied for its efficacy and economy for decades. Chiropractors are more than just neck and back doctors. They can help not only with your headaches but so much more.

Chiropractors have more education in nutrition, anatomy, differential diagnostics, and imaging than medical doctors. A medical doctor's education is filled with pharmacology, which chiropractors study minimally.[11]

When you seek medical treatment, a medical doctor typically treats you with a drug, whereas a chiropractor can help you find a way to become well without using medication to mute your symptoms.

Treatment of Headache Disorders: A systematic review of randomized clinical trials." *Cephalalgia.*
Roland Bryans, DC, et al., "Evidence-Based Guidelines for the Chiropractic Treatment of Adults With Headache." *Journal of Manipulative & Physiological Therapeutics.*
[11] Jensen, Your Chiropractic Wellness (blog). "Chiropractic Education vs. Medical Education."

There is a reason medicine requires a prescription. I have had many patients who suffered terribly after taking just a few doses of a new medication prescribed by their doctor. Some of their more common side effects have included chronic pain, hormone imbalance, weight gain, and depression.

Serious negative side effects are real and do occur. This is why I strongly believe that if you have the time to see if the natural route works for you, pursue it. Medicine is better suited for critical ailments, when you do not have the time to allow your body to heal itself. To use medicine for anything else is unhealthy in the long run.

If you can get better with chiropractic treatment and lifestyle changes, those approaches are better than turning to a pain pill. If you go the prescription route for pain, you are not solving the problem. You're masking it and allowing the pain to worsen with time while the pain medication's efficacy wanes over time.

If you suffer from headaches, chiropractors can help you determine the type of headache you are suffering from and the cause of it. They will treat you and/or refer you to a different healthcare practitioner if necessary. They can also teach you what you can do to naturally alleviate headaches.

I look forward to a time when patients try chiropractic first to see if it can help (knowing their chiropractor will send them to a medical doctor or surgeon if they feel their condition is beyond what chiropractic can alleviate). Even if chiropractic does not work for you, you can always fall back on the medical route. But if you start with the medical route, especially surgery, sometimes there is no turning back.

I believe if people saw a chiropractor before going to a medical doctor, it would solve a lot of our healthcare problems in America (both the costs of healthcare and the general health of this country).

I love that I am married to a chiropractor. He can help keep my spine flexible and youthful. My goal is to feel well until I am at least 102 years old. I would say 120 years old, since some studies suggest that humans are genetically designed to live that long, [12] but we live on a polluted planet and I am not perfect…which is a good thing. Attempting to be perfect is too stressful, and remember, stress leads to dis-ease, which leads to disease and early death.

---

[12] Ruiz-Torres and W. Beier, "On Maximum Human Life Span: Interdisciplinary approach about its limits." *Advances in Gerontology.* 16 (2005)

Chapter 25 : CHIROPRACTIC MANIPULATION: WHAT IS IT, HOW CAN IT HELP, AND IS IT SAFE?

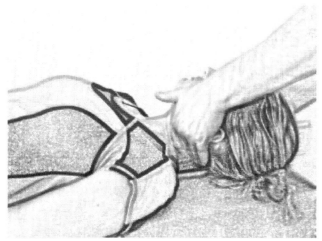

Figure 25-1

I MAY BE BIASED, but I believe that chiropractic manipulation to the cervical spine and cranial bones are the best treatments for most types of headaches (Figure 25-1). Especially since it is super safe! It also often results in more health benefits than expected. Bonus! In this chapter, I explain the how and why. I hope this information encourages you to try chiropractic if you haven't already.

What Is a Chiropractic Manipulation?

During a chiropractic manipulation (also called an adjustment), a chiropractor applies a high-velocity, short-lever arm thrust to a bone to decompress a joint, restoring normal motion to the joint and/or normal alignment of the bones. Let me explain, in layman's terms, how a chiropractor does an adjustment.

To perform an adjustment, the chiropractor introduces a quick stretch to the muscles surrounding a joint while staying within the joint's normal range of motion.

Muscles have a quick stretch reflex, and when a muscle is stretched quickly, nerves in the muscle respond by causing the muscle to relax. This autonomic reflex protects the muscles from tearing during any quick stretch.

A chiropractic adjustment does not go nearly deep enough to risk tearing muscles, but the nerves and muscles do not know this. All they know is that an external force is making the muscles stretch quickly, so the nerves protect the muscle from such external forces. Therefore, an adjustment causes muscles to relax.

Fluid is present in the space between the bones. When a chiropractor performs a quick stretch, the barometric pressure of the joint fluid decreases. Like any fluid, decreasing the pressure causes the release of gasses (in this case, oxygen, nitrogen, and carbon dioxide).

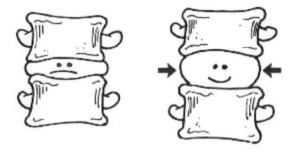

Figure 25-2

An everyday example of this phenomenon is when you open a can of soda. A soda can is under pressure, and when you open it, the barometric pressure of the fluid decreases, and bubbles come out of the liquid. A joint, however, is a closed "container," so the "bubble(s)" pop immediately.

Why an Adjustment Helps

Many amazing physiological events that facilitate healing occur with an adjustment. Examples of these physiological events are:

Increases Range of Motion

During an adjustment, a chiropractor moves a joint within its full healthy range of motion. It is safe because the chiropractor is far from overstretching the ligaments. If you do not move enough, joints degenerate. When is the last time you stretched all of your joints to their full range of motion? There is a reason we say, "If you don't use it, you lose it."

People stiffen as they get older not because of their chronological age, but because of their lack of stretching over time. Look at yogis. There are 100-year-old yogis who are more flexible than average middle-aged Americans.

I like to say that chiropractic manipulations are like going to a partner yoga class, but with a skilled partner who knows how to get to the end range of all your joints quickly and safely. Chiropractic adjustment is like yoga with an "oomph."

Reverses the Degenerative Process

Bones and joints are not rods of iron that rust with time. They are living tissue that degenerates with aberrant stressors over time. As you age, your ability to heal slows down, so you feel your body slowly lose the battle of healing. Everyday activities result in micro trauma to tissues.

When you are young, you heal rapidly because the joints are plump with nutrient-filled fluid, which is why you do not feel this micro trauma occurring. Over time, aberrant stressors of our modern lifestyle cause the joint fluid to slowly seep out, and the cells inside to start to die. With less nutrient-filled fluid and fewer cells to repair the damage as we age, each of these injuries is felt more profoundly. You take longer to heal, and the micro traumas begin to accumulate. This results in degeneration and arthritic changes.

But movement can help heal this damage. It was once thought that cartilage in the joints just wears away with time. Now we know there are cells (chondrocytes) inside each joint that repair the cartilage. Unfortunately, most people cause damage faster than the few chondrocytes can fix it, resulting in degeneration.

We need movement to support the cell repair and to facilitate the flow of nutrients in and waste out required for the repair process. Why?

Blood delivers nutrients to the joints, but for the nutrients to seep into the joint fluid, the joint fluid has to stir. Movement stirs the joint fluid and allows blood in the capillary bed to deliver nutrients deeper inside the joint fluid. The cells inside the joints receive the nutrients they need for this rebuilding process. Thus, simply moving your joints helps them heal.

If you sit too long, you are literally "starving" your joints. The weight of your body slowly squishes the fluid out of them (Figure 25-3). If joints do not have fluid flowing in with much-needed nutrients, the joints will degenerate over time.

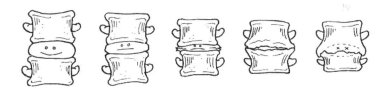

Figure 25-3: Discs degenerating over time (not a cause of age, but a co-factor)

Like physical movement, an adjustment literally "feeds" the joints it moves. When the gas bubbles form in the joint and pop, the fluid stirs and nutrients flow in, facilitating the healing of the joints and reversing the degenerative process (Figure 25-4).

Chiropractic Adjustment

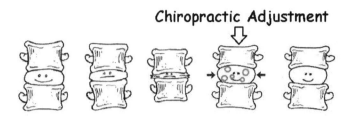

Figure 25-4: Chiropractic adjustment decompressing a joint, reversing the degenerative process

The increased space between the bones takes the pressure off of the nerves (decreasing one's experience of pain) and allows for more blood flow and lymphatic drainage. All of this facilitates the healing of the surrounding tissues.

Even young adults who do not move enough will experience degeneration in their joints. I am seeing people at younger ages getting degenerative joint disease from sitting too much beginning early in their life.

Relaxes Spastic Muscles

An adjustment relaxes spastic muscles through the quick stretches I described earlier in the chapter.

This is why adjusting the neck (cervical spine) helps with tension headaches. One quick adjustment relaxes the neck muscles far more than a whole hour of massage. A cervical adjustment is far safer than taking pain medication in the long run, and it corrects the cause of the head pain, unlike pain medication that just masks the pain.

Healing Occurs, Even at a Biochemical Level

During an adjustment, other biochemical reactions occur. The body releases endorphins into the area of the adjustment. This provides the short-term pain relief people report after an adjustment. The long-term effects of an adjustment are a faster healing rate and a restoration of full range of motion.

Chiropractic Adjustments Are Safe

I have patients who come in very concerned about getting their neck adjusted, despite being, in my opinion, one of the best treatments for headache sufferers. Unfortunately, these patients have heard that neck adjustments can cause paralysis or strokes.

If a patient has paralysis or a stroke after seeing a chiropractor, then that patient was at risk of paralysis or stroke from any regular activities of daily living. An adjustment does not move the neck outside of the normal range of motion. For something terrible to go wrong, the neck had to have an abnormality that made the patient vulnerable with any kind of movement. Tilting the head back to wash their hair could cause as much injury.

Just by living you are at risk of having a stroke. I have adjusted the necks of several thousand patients dozens, if not hundreds, of times to date. That is tens, if not hundreds, of thousands of neck adjustments I have personally performed. Every one of my patients feels an increase of motion, and most feel an immediate relief of pain after a neck adjustment. Not one of my adjustments has resulted in a stroke, let alone paralysis.

In fact, you are just as likely to have an adverse vascular event within twenty-four hours of seeing your regular doctor as when seeing your chiropractor.[13] Either you are going to have a stroke or not. Sadly, if it happens after seeing your chiropractor, some people want to blame the chiropractor.

Even medical organizations can't deny that chiropractic adjustments are safe.[14]

You are more likely to be struck by lighting (1 per 0.96 million lightning strikes)[15] in any given year than to be seriously hurt by a manipulation to the neck (1 per 1.565 million manipulations).

Research validates that chiropractic manipulation is much safer than taking NSAIDs.[16] Yet people in our culture are generally more comfortable taking a pain pill than having a neck manipulation! I believe this is due to misinformation. In fact, people *die daily* due to medicine taken as prescribed. Yet most people feel comfortable taking their medications!

---

[13] Cassidy, et al., "Risk of Vertebrobasilar Stroke and Chiropractic Care: Results of a population-based case-control and case-crossover study." *Spine.*

[14] "Chiropractic adjustment." Mayo Clinic.

[15] "How Dangerous is Lightning?" National Weather Service.

[16] Blower, et al., "Emergency Admissions for Upper Gastrointestinal Disease and Their Relation to NSAIDs Use." *Alimentary Pharmacology and Therapeutics.*
Fries, et al., "Toward an Epidemiology of Gastropathy Associated with Nonsteroidal Anti-inflammatory Drug Use." *Gastroenterology.*

Even the "Side Effects" of Spinal Manipulation Are Often Beneficial

The health benefits of an adjustment are often greater than expected. By stretching the vertebrae of the spine apart and creating more space for the nerves that exit the spinal cord, blood flow and lymph drainage increase. This allows nutrients to flow into and waste to flow out of the tissues, resulting in ideal conditions for the tissues to not only heal, but to function optimally. Without this space, there is more pressure on the nerves, blood vessels, and tissues.

Nerves especially do not like pressure; they function better with space. Better communication between the brain (vs. mind) and the body makes for better functioning organs, leading to a healthier body in general. This is why patients often report their headaches resolve, their sinuses drain, and/or the pressure in their ears clears after a neck adjustment. These are all great side effects for those suffering from head pain. This is why I love chiropractic.

Nerves that exit the neck region send signals to the head and upper extremities. So if these nerves are being compressed, they will cause head, neck, arm, or hand pain (Figure 25-5 and 25-6).

189

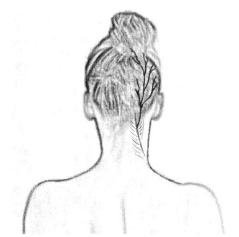

Figure 25-5: Neck adjustments take pressure off the nerves that exit the neck region, often providing relief from headaches

After treating neck pain with a cervical (neck) adjustment, I often hear things like "I haven't had a migraine since," "My sinuses have cleared," "My vertigo is gone," "My carpal tunnel syndrome resolved," and "My arms don't fall asleep or hurt anymore."

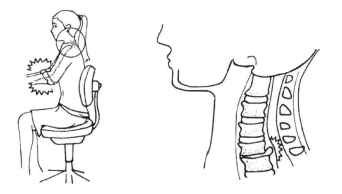

Figure 25-6: Example of a nerve being pinched in the neck, resulting in arm pain, numbness, tingling, and/or weakness, explaining why adjusting the neck can help alleviate arm pain

Nerves that exit the mid-back region send signals to the organs in the mid torso, including the lungs, stomach, spleen, and liver. After treating for mid-back pain, I have heard things like "My GERD has improved" and "My asthma is better."

Nerves that exit the lower back region of the spine send signals to the organs in the lower torso, including the lower intestines, reproductive organs, and lower extremities. After treating lower back pain, I often hear things like "My bowel movements have been more regular than ever," "My menstrual cycle is more normal," "My ED (erectile dysfunction) seems to have resolved," and "I was told by my medical doctor that I was infertile, and now I am pregnant!"

After treating children, their parents report, "They are calmer," "They are sleeping better," and "They are able to focus more."

I prefer these types of "side effects" to the side effects people experience with allopathic medicine, which often have incredibly long lists of possible negative side effects, including "Can cause death." When you take any medicine, there is always some negative effect; sometimes that negative effect ends up outweighing the benefit.

In nearly two decades of treating patients, I can't tell you how many people have reported that their head pain resolved after just a few treatments, even after suffering for years and spending thousands of dollars on specialists but seeing no improvement.

Finding Headache Relief with Chiropractic after Twenty Years of Pain

A recent extreme case was a patient in her thirties who had suffered daily headaches since she was eight years old. On a good day, the pain was tolerable and she could work; but at least once a week, she was bedridden with pain. Like many of my other chronic headache patients, she had seen specialists all over the country and had spent thousands of dollars. Each specialist offered her pain medications and/or muscle relaxers. Not one helped her determine the cause of her pain. Not one suggested trying chiropractic.

The pain was crippling her and grossly affecting the quality of her life. She was missing more and more work as the severity and frequency of her pain increased. Her boss was my patient and asked me if I thought I could help.

I told the boss that, at worst, I could help the employee find someone who could help her, and at best, I would help her. The pain-ridden woman was ready to try anything—even a treatment like chiropractic, which she considered alternative and not likely to help her because she had seen a chiropractor years before. Her previous chiropractic treatments had provided relief, but only temporarily (relief lasting only a few days). Now, her headaches were even worse, so she was doubtful chiropractic could help her.

I assured her that I would do more than just adjust her; I would help her determine the root cause of her headaches. I also explained that I had had success with other sufferers of chronic daily headaches.

Desperate, she agreed to give me a try.

After taking a history and conducting a physical examination, I told her she was likely suffering from both migraine and tension headaches. I was sure I could help with the tension, but the migraine headaches would take some lifestyle modifications. She agreed to try both.

The first adjustment to her cervical spine (neck) and cranium (skull) gave her a couple hours of relief, and her next headache was not as intense. After three treatments, she reported four consecutive days without any head pain. She started a diet diary and followed a rotation diet.

Now she gets mild headaches only during her menstrual cycle. These headaches are short in duration, lasting less than a few hours. She no longer needs her prescription pain medication. Only rarely does she need to take an over-the-counter pain reliever. When she does need one, the pill actually works for her, whereas before, even a prescription-strength dose would barely dull the pain.

She no longer misses work and is enjoying life on a whole new level. For the first time, she was able to go on a trip out of the country because she felt safe to be far from her doctors and prescription medications. This is yet another reason why I love my job.

Determining Whether Neck Manipulation Is Right for You

I hope the information in this chapter has helped persuade you to see a chiropractor to determine if a neck adjustment is an appropriate treatment for your headaches.

If you are going to receive a manipulation, simply ask how many manipulations your chiropractor performs on a weekly basis. Ask how successful they are at treating headaches. Also ask if they do cranial (head) manipulation because that often relieves headaches as well. The answers to these questions will help you figure out how skilled and practiced the chiropractor is at treating your condition.

You can also seek treatments for your headaches from other healthcare providers, including acupuncturists, massage therapists, physical therapists, doctors of osteopathy, and other body-moving practitioners. It often takes a village of healers to help you combat your headaches.

So how do you go about finding a healthcare provider? I explain that in the next chapter.

Chapter 26 : WHAT TO LOOK FOR IN A PRACTITIONER

HOW DO YOU FIND a practitioner or a group of healers (be it a chiropractor, medical doctor, massage therapist, physical therapist, osteopath, naturopath, acupuncturist, or any other type of healer) to help you treat your headaches? This is a loaded question, but the following are my two cents of advice.

First, find your practitioners by asking friends and family for referrals. The web is a good place to find out more about a practitioner, but it is not the best place to choose one. Anyone can look good online and put in fake testimonials. Try to use sites like www.yelp.com where people can post good and bad reviews without the business owners cherry-picking only the good reviews. This will increase the likelihood of getting legitimate evaluations.

Try to find people who have seen the specific practitioner and ask yourself these questions when you visit the practitioner yourself:

Does the Practitioner Really Listen to You?

Sadly, many in the medical field are in it for the wrong reason, or their reasons do not match your needs. You need to find a practitioner who has a passion for helping their patients. One indicator of this is how much they listen to their patients during an appointment. Most proper diagnoses come from taking an accurate history and getting a complete description of the current symptoms. Most physical examination, imaging, and laboratory work is performed to verify the diagnosis, not to find the problem.

Unfortunately, many doctors get burned out because of the fiasco that is the current political and insurance landscape. They are forced to see more people in less time and are required to complete vastly more paperwork and coding of a patient's symptoms. Eventually, many practitioners end up shutting down emotionally, closing off their humanity in order to survive going through the motions expected of them.

Doctors are people too, but you should not place the doctor's needs above your own when seeking treatment. Find a doctor whom you like on a personal level and who genuinely seems to care for you. This will positively affect your healing.

Does the Practitioner Give You the Time You Need?

Understand that more time does not necessarily mean a greater quality of care. If the practitioner is efficient and very good, they will not need as much time, but you should feel like you received their full attention and a full treatment when you are with them. You should feel that you got what you needed. I always end my treatments by asking my patients if I took care of everything, or if there is something else they need. This assures me I covered what they came in for, and if I did not, this gives the patient the opportunity to express their needs.

Sometimes I just need a few minutes to treat my patient; other times I end up spending a whole hour. It makes scheduling tough, but the rare times my patients have to wait, they know it was not because I overbooked but because someone needed more time. My patients appreciate that I give extra time if needed, and they recognize that someday it may be they who need that extra time.

Has the Practitioner Helped You? How Many Treatments Did it Take? How Much Did it Cost?

Ask the practitioner at the beginning whether your aliment is something they understand, have experience with, and have had success treating in the past. What do they think your prognosis is? Will they be able to treat you within a reasonable budget?

If the treatment is costly, maybe you can find a cheaper fix while still maintaining the quality of care. Costlier does not necessarily mean higher quality care. Beware, however, that you sometimes get what you pay for. Do not shortchange the quality of your healthcare to the point of negatively affecting your health.

If the practitioner does not think you have a good prognosis, don't waste your time or money on them! If your prognosis was bad, that is simply an opinion of someone who has not routinely seen success with your ailment. Find a different practitioner, one who has had success with your ailment, so they can give you a better prognosis.

For example, I have had patients who were told by several practitioners that they would never be able to turn their head fully left or right ever again because they had worn a neck collar for months after having broken their neck bones. When you stabilize joints, such as by wearing a collar, you prevent movement. Like the old saying goes, "If you don't use it, you lose it."

Accordingly, when their doctor had them finally remove the collar, they ended up with an immobile, very stiff neck. Many of these post-neck-fracture patients completed a course of physical therapy, which helped loosen up the neck somewhat by stretching the muscles. Even so, these patients were still severely limited by the immobilized joints in the neck.

Some of these patients were told by their medical doctors never to try chiropractic. I find it interesting that a medical doctor who is not trained in a technique like chiropractic feels qualified to restrict a patient from choosing that treatment option. I would never tell a patient that they should not take a medicine because that is not in my scope of practice. With that said, I have had many allopathic doctors suggest chiropractic to their patients.

I have also had patients who were informed by another chiropractor that they could not get an adjustment because they had a history of having a broken neck and their joint planes were no longer normal (because their bones remodeled aberrantly).

Thankfully, all of these people had friends or family members who knew me. Their friends or family members told them that they should at least consult with me, if for no other reason to get my opinion. I need only a few minutes to examine the neck to tell if I can help them.

My goal with these cases is to be able to see within six visits some improvement in the range of motion of their neck, which is often limited to about 10 degrees of movement. My second goal is to have their neck moving over 50 degrees within the next six visits (70 degrees is considered within normal range, but 50 degrees is more functional than what they typically start with after months of wearing a collar). If the patient is responding, as my past experience suggests they should, then their outcome should be as successful as my previous patients with similar injuries.

If people are going to spend their health dollars on a treatment, that treatment should have a favorable outcome. To help determine whether progress is being made, measurements should be taken incrementally during the course of the treatments to show objectively whether the patient is responding favorably. If there is no measurable improvement partway through the treatment, then the condition needs to be reexamined. You may be getting treatment for the wrong condition. You cannot keep doing the same treatment and expect a different result.

I have had multiple patients come see me after their previous chiropractor failed to make them feel better after dozens of treatments. I was glad these patients were willing to suspend blame on the tool of chiropractic. With my chiropractic skills, I was able to help them feel better after just a few treatments. The rare times I cannot help a patient, I direct them to health practitioners who can.

It is important to find a practitioner who is willing and able to be your partner in obtaining optimal health. That practitioner should know their limitations and whether the treatment options for you go beyond their abilities. If they are not willing to be your partner, they are unlikely to help you reach optimal health. When a practitioner reaches their limitation in being able to help you, that is their limitation, not necessarily your limitation on being able to get well.

Think of all the aliments that used to be considered untreatable. They were not truly untreatable, but instead were outside the abilities of medical care at the time. These same ailments *are* treatable today because of the increase in medical knowledge. Unfortunately, we healthcare providers may not know the treatment you need, even if a treatment is currently available for you.

It reminds me of the old joke, "Do you know what they call the person who graduated at the bottom of his class at medical school? Doctor." Just because one doctor, or one type of healthcare practitioner, cannot see how to help you solve your problem, it does not mean your problem is unsolvable.

Are They Open to You Seeing Other Practitioners?

I always welcome other practitioners' views on my patients' wellness. Not just from specialists in other fields, but from other chiropractors as well. Everyone brings something unique to the table, and sometimes new eyes bring new perspectives. I have a dozen patients who see other chiropractors for treatments I do not offer or because the other chiropractor is more convenient (closer to their work or home); these patients see me only when their treatments are not helping as expected and they need another opinion. Some patients simply like to have a relationship with multiple chiropractors so they are more likely to be seen in a timely manner.

I encourage all of my patients to see a variety of other health practitioners (medical doctors, acupuncturists, massage therapists, physical therapists, etc.). At a minimum, these other practitioners confirm my diagnosis and treatments. If they do not confirm it, then it prompts me to reexamine the problem more deeply. This can provide a learning experience for me and further confirmation for the patient. Or the patient may have two different opinions and more information to bring to a third practitioner to find the root of the problem. In either case, the collaboration is more helpful than the Lone Ranger approach.

I cannot tell you how many times patients have come to me after seeing several doctors, each of whom gave the patient a different diagnosis. I examine the patient and review what has already been done so I can help them determine the root cause and so they can figure out their next step toward wellness.

I once had a patient who was seeing a surgeon and physical therapist for his knee and shoulder. I was only working on his back because of the politics of worker's compensation. The patient was a quiet, stout man—not one to complain. The surgeon saw the patient after the patient's physical therapy sessions ended, and after asking him a few questions, the surgeon released the patient to go back to work without even physically examining him!

The poor patient could not raise his left arm above 90 degrees (180 degrees is considered normal), and he couldn't stand for more than an hour without excruciating pain. The patient was understandably concerned. He knew he could not do his labor-intensive job.

I asked the patient if he had explained this to his surgeon. He did not tell the surgeon because the surgeon did not ask him the right questions. When the patient was asked if he was in pain, he replied no because he was just sitting in the examination room, not feeling too bad. After a couple more leading questions, the surgeon deemed that he was ready to return to work without even touching him, let alone examining him!

I explained to the patient that if the surgeon knew of his limitations and the true level of his pain, he would not be released to go back to work. I advised him to get another opinion. Thankfully, he did.

The second surgeon approved an MRI of his shoulder, which revealed several muscle tears. This surgeon also reexamined the patient's knee and found it to be far from well. So the second surgeon scheduled shoulder surgery and prescribed more physical therapy for the patient's knee.

If the patient had not sought out that second opinion, he would have had to return to work still broken, and who knows what kind of long-term effects the further damage would have caused. The moral of this story is, the more educated people on your team, the better.

Sadly, I have many more of these types of stories. I even have had health practitioners tell their patients not to see other practitioners. I have had several patients who were told by their physical therapists not to see me because seeing both a chiropractor and physical therapist was "the same thing" and that it would be "fraudulent" to bill insurance for two of the same. I believe this is a sign of their own insecurities, not a sign of a practitioner who has your best interests at heart.

You have the right to see as many healing professionals as you need to in order to get to the core of your condition. Each type of practitioner (and maybe even each individual practitioner) will have their own individual technique to offer. If nothing else, they can help verify that you are receiving the right kind of treatment.

If you receive satisfactory answers to the first four questions, then after seeing the provider, ask yourself the following questions:

Are They Actually Helping You?

Do their treatments hurt? Some therapists have a "no pain, no gain" mentality, resulting in treatments that may be more painful than they need to be.

If you feel like your healthcare provider (be it massage or physical therapist, chiropractor, acupuncturist, or any other practitioner) is hurting you, even if they are not, your belief that they are hurting you will impair your healing. This phenomenon is called "the negative placebo effect."

I always tell my patients to listen to their instincts. If what I do or say does not jive with them, they should tell me. Their instinct always trumps my recommendation or technique. It just means we have to find another technique that works for them, both physically and mentally. You cannot separate the two.

Many of my patients say that, for such a small female, I give a mighty adjustment and dig deep with my soft-tissue work. But many patients receive ultra-gentle care from me. I cater my treatment to the patient's needs and limitations. I am not going to adjust a construction worker the same as I would an elderly lady with osteopenia.

There are times where I am pressing on tender muscles, but I aim to produce good pain. My patients understand that it may hurt in the moment, but the body knows it is a good hurt and a productive movement toward wellness. I never want to cause bad pain. That, to me, is a pressure that causes more harm than good, such as bruising healthy tissues. I aim to mobilize joints, not strain them.

This is where the art of practice comes into play. Anyone can move a joint, but not everyone can move it safely and well, in a manner that that patient is comfortable with. That is why such practices take years of education and requires licensure.

Is the Practitioner Living Up to Your Expectations?

At your first appointment, a practitioner should give you a rough timeline of when you should start seeing results, how likely you will recover and to what degree. If you are not seeing the results as expected, get another opinion. Do not be afraid to seek more than one healer's advice, to validate the root cause of your pain.

When a patient isn't seeing results as expected, it can be due to the provider not treating you completely, or a misdiagnosis resulting in the wrong treatment being prescribed.

My least favorite thing is when a patient comes in with what I call a "garbage can diagnosis," which is basically a fancy combination of Latin words that describe their symptoms but not any underlying causes or conditions. Then, armed with this "diagnosis," a medical doctor will generally attempt to cover up the patient's symptoms with drugs. It is relatively easy to do, and everyone is happy at the cessation of symptoms. But the long-term cost of this approach is immeasurable: The patient's health will continue to deteriorate over time because no one is addressing the root of the problem.

To make matters worse, the effectiveness of any medicine decreases over time as the body learns to break it down. This reduced effectiveness results in having to increase the dose over time. Sadly, the patient is trained to blame this problem on the fact that they are aging. No! The patient needs to learn what the root of the problem is so they can properly treat it and so their body can start healing over time instead of worsening.

I love my job. Every day I get to watch people transform from the belief that their health was naturally going to worsen with time to a place where their lives and abilities actually *improve* over time. I have many patients who are healthier in their forties and fifties than they were in their twenties and thirties.

Good luck creating your optimal healing team!

TRIAD OF WELLNESS
For Headaches

Sleep Well
Relax & Meditate

Move Well
Exercise & Stretch often,
Release Trigger &
Pressure points

Eat & Drink Well
Avoid Triggers &
Stay Hydrated!

In Conclusion . . .

If your headaches are not due to some underlying disease, using some, if not all, of the techniques I've included in this book should reduce or eliminate the need to take pain-relieving medication for a headache.

On the rare occasion you still need a pain pill or shot, it should work even better for you because your body will not have built up a tolerance to the remedy.

I hope this book has been informative and will enable you to be more collaborative with your professional healthcare providers so you can plan your path to a pain-free and healthy life.

If I have helped you, I have fulfilled my mission in writing this book. I am writing my Combat Dis-Ease Series—each book a message in a bottle I send out in a sea of confusing and conflicting information—with the hope that they contain the map that helps you find your way to wellness.

Wishing you the best of health,

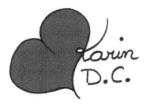

Karin Drummond, DC

Quick Reference for Basic Trigger Points, Pressure Points, and Stretches for Headaches

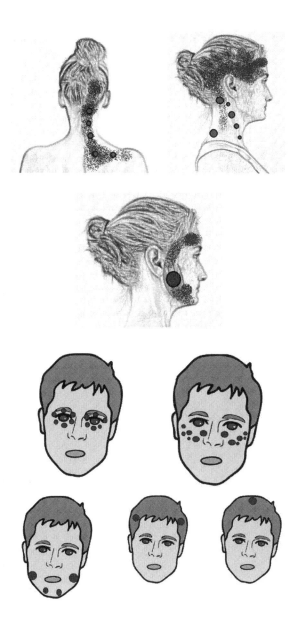

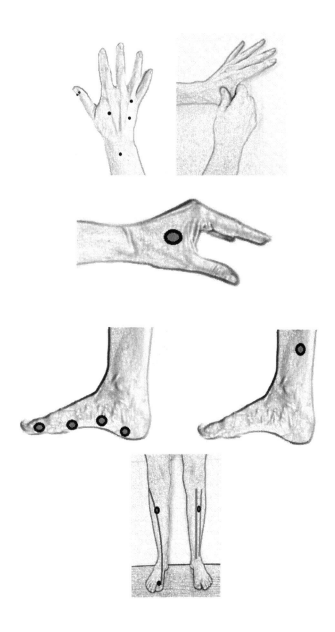

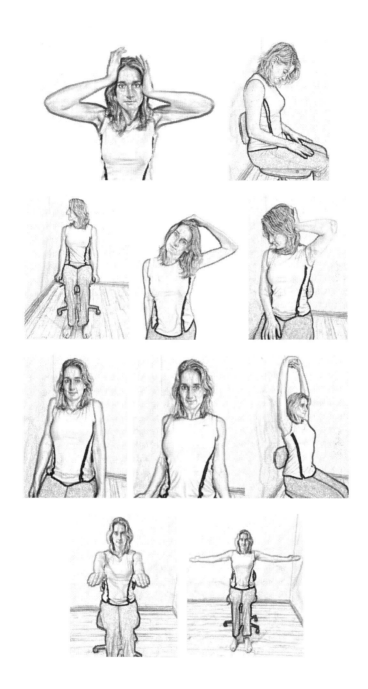

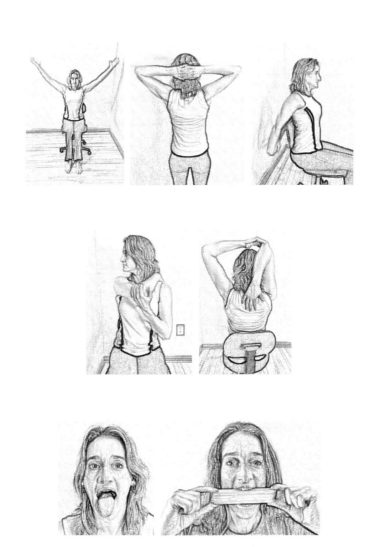

References

American Gastroenterological Association. "Study Shows Long-term Use of NSAIDs Causes Severe Intestinal Damage." ScienceDaily. www.sciencedaily.com/releases/2005/01/050111123706.htm.

American Headache Society. "REM Sleep Deprivation Plays a Role in Chronic Migraine." ScienceDaily (June 23, 2010). www.sciencedaily.com/releases/2010/06/100623085528.htm.

Astin, J.A. and E. Ernst. "The Effectiveness of Spinal Manipulation for the Treatment of Headache Disorders: A systematic review of randomized clinical trials." *Cephalalgia* 22, no. 8 (2002): 617–623.

Blower, Al, A. Brooks, C.G. Fenn, A. Hill, M.Y. Pearce, S. Morant, and K.D. Bardhan. "Emergency Admissions for Upper Gastrointestinal Disease and Their Relation to NSAIDs Use." *Alimentary Pharmacology and Therapeutics* 11, no. 2 (1997): 283–91.

Boyles, Salynn. "Low-Carb Diets Improve Cholesterol Long Term." WebMD Health News. (August 2, 2010) http://www.webmd.com/cholesterol-management/news/20100802/low-carb-diets-improve-cholesterol-long-term.

Heiman ML1, Greenway FL2.A healthy gastrointestinal microbiome is dependent on dietary diversity. Mol Metab. 2016 Mar 5;5(5):317-20. doi: 10.1016/j.molmet.2016.02.005. eCollection 2016.

Bryans, R., M. Descarreaux M, Duranleau, H. Marcoux, B. Potter, R. Ruegg, L. Shaw, R. Watkin, and E. White. "Evidence-based Guidelines for the Chiropractic Treatment of Adults with Headache." *Journal of Manipulative and Physiological Therapeutics* 34, no. 5 (June 2011): 274-89. doi:10.1016/j.jmpt.2011.04.008.

Cassidy, J.D., E. Boyle, P. Côté, Y. He, S. Hogg-Johnson, F.L. Silver, S.J. Bondy. "Risk of Vertebrobasilar Stroke and Chiropractic Care: Results of a population-based case-control and case-crossover study." *Spine* 33 (4 Suppl) (2008): S176–83.

Fernández, MD, Ernesto. *Headache: The Journal of Head and Face Pain* 30, no. 3

Fries, J.F., S.R. Miller, P.W. Spitz, C.A Williams, H.B. Hubert, and D.A. Bloch. "Toward an Epidemiology of Gastropathy Associated with Nonsteroidal Anti-inflammatory Drug Use." *Gastroenterology* 96 (1989): 647–655.

Jensen, Paul. Your Chiropractic Wellness (blog). "Chiropractic Education vs. Medical Education." http://yourchiropracticwellness.com/tag/chiropractic-education-vs-medical-education.

Mayo Clinic. "Chiropractic adjustment." Last updated August 13, 2015. www.mayoclinic.org/tests-procedures/chiropractic-adjustment/basics/risks/prc-20013239.

National Weather Service. "How Dangerous is Lightning?" www.lightningsafety.noaa.gov/odds.shtml.

Ruiz-Torres, A. and W. Beier. "On Maximum Human Life Span: Interdisciplinary approach about its limits." *Advances in Gerontology* 16 (2005): 14–20. www.ncbi.nlm.nih.gov/pubmed/16075672.

University of Maryland Medical Center. "Migraine headaches." Last reviewed September 29, 2015. http://umm.edu/health/medical/altmed/condition/migraine-headache#ixzz3axxDHytg.

Vicodin Addiction. "Nearly 100 Percent of the World's Vicodin Prescriptions are Used in U.S." www.addictionvicodin.com/addiction-news/all-the-worlds-vicodin-prescriptions-in-united-states/.

Zimmerman, H.J. "Drugs Used to Treat Rheumatic and Musculospastic Disease," in *Hepatotoxicity: The adverse effects of drugs and other chemicals on the liver.* 2nd ed. Philadelphia: Lippincott, 1999.

ABOUT THE AUTHOR

Karin Drummond, DC, lives in Bloomington, Indiana. She graduated with distinction from the University of Victoria with a bachelor of science degree. She finished the four-year doctorate of chiropractic degree at the University of Western States in 2000. She moved to her husband's hometown of Bloomington, Indiana, and has practiced there ever since. She now calls it home, living at its edge in the country with her husband and two children. She has been voted her town's number one chiropractor seven times as of 2016.

Passionate about living well, she keeps up with new research in the health field and practices what she preaches. Her patients have told her for years that she needed to write a book because she is such a great source of information on healthy living. Once she discovered how easy it was to publish a book, she decided to take advantage of this medium to help spread her thoughts on living well. Her first book, *Top Seven Ways to Combat the Effects of Sitting,* was published in 2015. This is her second book, and she is planning on publishing many more books on a variety of topics.

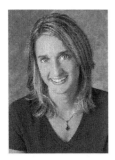

www.drummondchiropractic.com

Other books by Dr. Karin Drummond

Top Seven Ways to Combat the Effects of Sitting: The Silent Killer

Up and coming books:

Combat Slouching:
A Chiropractor's advice for those who suffer with aches, pains, stiffness, spinal deformities like hyperkyphosis and other effects of slouching.

Combat Irritable Bowel Syndrome:
A chiropractor's advice for those who suffer with diarrhea, constipation, spastic gallbladder, inflammation of the bowels, and other causes of abdominal pain.

Whiplash:
A Chiropractor's Journey from Whiplash to Wellness

and many other books to come…
All to help you find your path to wellness.

To find out more, visit her website
www.drummondchiropractic.com

Made in the USA
Middletown, DE
24 April 2019